# Eat to Heal

## A Surgeon's Guide to
## Nutrition and Wound Healing

Joseph F. McCaffrey MD FACS

# CONTENTS

# INTRODUCTION

Let's call her Mary. She was like many people we see at the wound care center. She was in her 80s and came to us because she had a rather large wound on her right leg directly over the shin bone. It just wasn't healing.

Mary hurt herself when she fell several weeks before she came to us. She was one of those feisty old women we all admire. Even though her family worried about her, she was still living on her own and actually doing quite well. In fact, she hurt her leg because she was still gardening. She fell when she was getting some tools out of her garden shed. She tripped and as she went down she hit her leg on the edge of a cinderblock, ripping the skin open.

This would have been a nasty injury in anyone. As a testimony to Mary's overall strength, she didn't break anything. However the edge of the cinder block really did a job on her thin skin and the soft tissue. It crushed and ripped off skin and the little fat underneath almost to the bone.

Immediately after the fall she went to urgent care. Later she followed up with her family doctor.

It wasn't the type of wound that could be stitched. The doctors cleaned it up and treated it with the usual ointments and dressings. At one point it looked infected and she had a course of antibiotics.

Despite this appropriate treatment, week after week went by and the wound wasn't getting any better. That's why she was referred to our wound center.

Working as a surgeon, I've been witnessing wounds healing for several decades now. Rather than taking the process for granted, it seems more miraculous to me all the time.

As science probes deeper into what has to happen to heal a wound, it's evident to me that our current knowledge has only scratched the surface of the everyday miracle known as wound healing.

Healing is so routine, so ordinary that we often take it for granted. That is, we take it for granted until it doesn't happen. That's the point at which we are asked to see people at the wound care center.

For the last few years I've changed the focus of my practice to work exclusively in a specialized wound care center. This center and others like it exists because in a small percentage of people wound healing doesn't progress as it should. We're there to do what we can to figure out what's wrong and help things along as best we can.

Our first job is to see if we can determine why the wound isn't healing. Healing is normal. If it doesn't happen it means something is wrong. Something is preventing normal healing. So the first question is: What's preventing things from progressing normally?

Often we will find something specific such as uncontrolled swelling, or diabetes, or kidney failure, or poor circulation, or...

But aside from these attention-getting items there are often less obvious factors contributing to poor healing. Major among these is poor nutrition.

The poor nutrition that we see isn't the wasting malnourishment and starvation of poor countries. It's more subtle than that. Rather, a surprising percentage of the people we see lack key nutrients in their diet. The sad fact is that the typical American diet is pretty poor at best. It doesn't take much to create a situation where wound healing just doesn't happen.

Mary was like many older people living alone. She didn't particularly enjoy cooking for herself, food didn't seem to taste as good anymore and she just didn't have much appetite. Her family reported that she "ate like a bird". Her diet wasn't awful, but it wasn't great either.

Anyone at 80 just doesn't heal as well as they did when they were 20 years old. They need all the help they can get, including a healthy diet.

We cleaned the wound well, saw her every week to remove dead tissue from it, used an advanced wound care dressing to minimize the bacteria in the wound and maintain optimum moisture levels (a Goldilocks approach is needed:

not too wet, not too dry). In addition, we applied a gentle compression wrap to control the swelling that was present.

These manipulations and techniques are the things we do at the center that get most of the attention. Using a scalpel to cut out dead tissue and applying a fancy dressing are obvious. However the less obvious step of encouraging healthy nutrition is equally important. In fact, as you'll see later in this book, if a person doesn't have the raw materials that good nutrition provides anything we do with the wound is unlikely to help. It certainly won't have maximum effectiveness.

We encourage all our patients to pay more attention to their diet. The exact recommendations depend on the person's situation and how much they are willing to do.

With Mary, we encouraged her to eat more regularly, with meals including lean protein and a variety of vegetables. Fortunately she had a supportive family that would help. Even so we thought it unlikely that she would get enough calories and protein from her diet alone so we recommended a nutritional supplement that included whey protein between meals. We also recommended a high potency multivitamin, omega 3 fats (in the form of fish oil capsules) and vitamin D.

I won't pretend that once we did these things healing was miraculously swift. It wasn't. However, within two weeks the wound that hadn't shown any improvement in two months was obviously getting better. Within a few more weeks, it was healed.

There's no one factor that's completely responsible for obtaining wound healing. It's a package deal. However, good nutrition is an important part of that package. In fact, it's the foundation and that foundation is what this book is about.

Here you'll discover the principles we use to guide the advice we give patients at the center. You'll discover that the nutritional guidelines that support wound healing are actually good for your health in general. We make adjustments when someone has a major wound, but overall the suggestions in this book are good advice for anyone. In fact, we frequently see family members making some changes in their own diet when they see the benefits in the person we are treating for a wound.

My hope is that the information here will help you be healthy and well, and if you should suffer from a wound, to heal it as swiftly as possible.

Joseph F. McCaffrey MD, FACS

# 1 LET FOOD BE YOUR MEDICINE

Let's begin with the obvious. We need food to live. Of course food has intense social and emotional implications, and I for one like to celebrate that. Like many, I consider sharing a good meal with family and friends to be one of the great joys in life.

But the focus here will be much more pragmatic. It will be more about food as a resource for our bodies and what we need to do to get the most out of that resource.

Some rather unromantic folks think of food almost solely as a source of energy. If we consider our body as an engine, then food is the biologic equivalent of fuel.

But even at a pragmatic level food is much more than that. Food isn't only fuel. Food provides the building blocks of our bodies. To continue the engine metaphor, food not only fuels the engine, it builds the car and engine in the first place.

In other words, food provides us with both the raw ingredients to construct our amazingly complex cells and organs and then the energy to keep things thriving.

Our bodies continually reconstruct and repair themselves. To again use the automotive metaphor, it's as if our cars not only use fuel to build and power the engine, they also gradually and continually rebuild the entire automobile as we drive.

This is why just eating a bunch of calories isn't enough. The quality of our diet plays a crucial role in determining our health and overall vitality.

Getting enough to eat hasn't always been easy. Throughout history most humans have spent a large portion of their lives struggling simply to get enough food to survive. The current epidemic of obesity suggests that getting enough to eat isn't as difficult today. Quantity is no longer an issue for most Americans.

Unfortunately, quality is another matter. The diet of most Americans is calorie rich but nutrient poor. Stand in any aisle of a grocery store and you see an astounding abundance of "food" but precious little of nutritional value.

While the obesity epidemic suggests that getting enough calories isn't a problem for most people in this country, the simultaneous epidemic of diet related diseases suggests that getting a proper mix of nutrients is a problem.

The bottom line: *if you want optimum health and vitality, you're going to need to think and act a little bit differently than most people. This is especially true if you have a wound to heal.*

In this short book, I intend to give you what I currently consider the principles of a healthy diet. I won't pretend that these are inviolate rules or the be all and end all. Over my 30 plus years in medicine I've had to reformulate what I believe to be healthy so many times that it keeps me humble now. These days I try not to be too dogmatic about my recommendations.

However, I have spent a good part of my life trying to understand what contributes to true wellness. I'm increasingly convinced that staying healthy doesn't have to be complicated. This is certainly true when it comes to diet.

We'll talk about things like glycemic index, insulin resistance, characteristics of different fats and so on but again: none of this has to be complicated.

Borrowing from a book I highly recommend ( In Defense of Food by Michael Pollan ), you can sum up the best dietary advice today in just a few words: "Eat real food. Not too much. Mostly plants."

Michael Pollan wrote In Defense of Food as a follow up to his book The Omnivore's Dilemma because after reading that book people kept asking him what kind of diet he recommended. The Omnivore's Dilemma examined the sources of food in today's world. Pollan begins with the premise that humans are omnivores meant to eat a range of food ( apologies to vegetarians but that's the way it is ). In The Omnivores Dilemma he examines in detail exactly where food comes from today and how it's handled.

After doing all that research, his practical advice came down to the seven words I just mentioned:


"Eat food. Not too much. Mostly plants."

Those seven words contain a lot of wisdom. In Defense of Food he expands on those words but it remains a short, entertaining, easy-to-read and thought provoking book. I highly recommend it.

If you want, you can stop reading now, follow that advice and do well. If you're interested in a bit more detail, read on...

I think it's helpful to consider diet at two levels: the overall big picture (the macro level) and the more detailed, nutrient specific level (the micro level).

On the overall level, our diet needs to provide us with both raw energy as well as the specific building blocks that a healthy metabolism demands.

The energy part of the equation is expressed as calories. In an ideal, balanced state we would be at a healthy weight with normal musculature and eat enough calories every day to go about our business doing whatever we want to do with plenty of energy and without a change in weight.

In this ideal state, the number of calories we eat matches the number of calories we need. We should have some body fat to serve as long-term emergency

5

energy storage, but this would be stable at less than 15 – 20% of body weight.

Still at the macro level, food is one of three things: carbohydrate, protein or fat. It's best to have a balance of all three.

Beyond raw calories, the nutrients in our food are critical. As I've stated, the sad fact is that most Americans are calorie rich but nutrient poor. The shelves in our grocery stores bulge with products providing calories without nutrition.

This is what Pollan alludes to with his phrase "eat food." He means eat real food, which he defines simply but effectively as something you're great-grandparents would recognize as food. Cheese-like substance squirted from a can? I don't think so.

Listen, I'm generally not one to bash businesses but much of the stuff offered by the food industry and heavily promoted by their ad agencies isn't doing us any good. It certainly doesn't provide nutrition. They sell it to make money, not to support your well-being. Even when they make health claims, those claims are almost always more of a marketing ploy than a statement of real benefits.

Enough of that rant...

A tremendous amount of research today focuses on compounds called phytonutrients – nutrients contained in plants. There are thousands of these compounds, many of which are proving to be exceptionally important for our health. I'll be telling you about some of these specifically later on, but first I want to give you some idea about why eating a wide variety of real foods is so important.

In this context, I'm using the term nutrient to refer to any naturally occurring compound in the food that the body uses as part of a metabolic process.

I won't even pretend to understand all the metabolic activities that take place simultaneously and continuously throughout our bodies. It's enough to know that all of these metabolic processes require appropriate raw materials as well as energy.

It's so complex I don't really think anyone can really get their mind around what's going on simultaneously. In medicine, we usually simplify it by focusing on one system at a time.

For example, one might study how digestion takes place beginning with food being chewed and the signals that go off to stimulate the release of saliva and initiate other digestive changes.

Swallowing requires coordinated muscular work. The act of chewing and swallowing triggers both nerve and hormonal signals that will further promote digestion.

The stomach lining releases a hormone (cholecystokinin) into the bloodstream which stimulates the gallbladder to contract at the right time to add bile to the digestive mix. At the same time, cells in the last part of the stomach release gastrin in just the right amount to stimulate other cells in the first part of the stomach to secrete acid.

I could go on and on, but this gives you an idea of just a few of the things that happen when you bite into a grilled cheese sandwich

And this is just one tiny part of digestion. There's a lot more going on in your G.I. tract while at the same time your immune system carries on constant surveillance and protection, your muscles move as you command, glands release hormones in precise amounts, the kidneys excrete waste products, your circulatory system delivers precisely the amount of blood each organ needs and on and on. It really is quite miraculous.

All of these activities require raw materials, the building blocks so-to-speak. There are only two sources of these raw materials: the air we breathe and the food we eat. That's it.

Let's try another metaphor. Imagine an extremely vibrant, prosperous and vital nation. This nation has a myriad of talented producers ranging from large corporations to small cottage industries to individual artisans. It has a complex distribution system that, when the raw materials are available, works beautifully to provide everything these multiple producers need to create their wonderful products on a just-in-time basis.

The weakness of this imaginary nation is that it <u>has to import all its raw materials</u>. It has none of its own. Things go wrong when something interferes with the steady supply of high-quality raw materials. Factories try to keep going with what's available, but the quality of manufactured goods plummets. Total output declines. Artisans are unable to do their best work. The overall vitality of the nation suffers.

Our bodies are an incredibly interconnected web of interacting physiologic activities with complexity beyond that of any industrialized nation. The body constantly forms and reforms itself. Even in a normal, healthy state the body continually produces new cells and there are an unfathomable number of biochemical processes all going continuously.

The body is marvelous and creative, but it can only work with what you give it. To use another metaphor, you can compare it to a master carpenter. If you give a master carpenter a limited number of crummy tools and poor quality, partially rotten wood he may be able to make something serviceable, but it will be nothing compared to what he could do given a beautifully equipped shop with the best raw materials imaginable.

You can think of the nutrients you supply your body in the same way. Optimum results require the best raw materials in the right amounts.

I mentioned that carbohydrates, proteins and fats provide energy. The building blocks of these energy sources (sugars, amino acids and fatty acids) also have metabolic roles. But our nutrient needs go far beyond this.

You're familiar with vitamins and minerals. However, it's increasingly clear that multiple other compounds beyond these exert a tremendous influence on our metabolism and our health. A key requirement of a healthy diet is that it not only provides calories (energy) but a wide range of nutrients as well.

Just getting enough calories, even with the right proportions between the three classes of macro nutrients, isn't enough. We need a wide array of micro nutrients as well. As a general rule, the greater the variety of foods we eat the better.

I'm sure you've heard the phrase "empty calories." That refers to calories without any accompanying nutrients. An obvious example is soft drinks (AKA soda or pop depending on where you live). Soda provides lots of calories from sugar, but no nutrients whatsoever.

Here is our goal. We want the right amount of calories from the right sources containing the widest variety of nutrients possible. How to go about doing that is the focus of this book.

We'll consider this in some detail. First we'll discuss that big picture I mentioned, the macro nutrients

11

(carbohydrates, proteins and fats). I'll explain ways of thinking about each of these that I find useful.

Then we'll look at things more closely. We'll consider what I call the micro level, the chemical nutrients your body requires. We emphasize some of the most crucial nutrients you need and what you can do to be sure that you're getting them.

We'll also discuss supplements that can be of help, especially with regards to wound healing.

I do recommend supplements, but always remember that the foundation has to be a sound diet. Supplements are just that: supplements. They can augment our diet but taking a bunch of pills, powders and capsules can never replace a healthy diet.

So let's get started. We'll begin with a basic question: How much food do we need?

# 2 HOW MUCH IS ENOUGH?

The crudest question about our diet is how much should we eat? How many calories do we need each day?

For most of humanity's history just getting enough to eat every day was a major chore. People often weren't successful.

Fortunately, today getting adequate calories is not an issue for virtually any American. Unfortunately, the quantity and quality of calories most people consume has given us an epidemic of obesity and diet related medical problems.

Diabetes, hypertension, heart disease, arthritis, stroke – all these and more have a strong dietary basis.

So what's the answer to the question: How many calories do we need?

The answer is "It depends." It depends on who we are and what we're doing. Nutritionists talk about basal metabolic rate as the starting point and then add calories according to an individual's unique energy needs.

13

The basal metabolic rate is the number of calories we need to live and carry out our bodies important basic functions (breathing, pumping blood, producing hormones, maintaining the immune system, etc.) when we're not doing much beyond sitting still. This is the minimum caloric intake a human needs to meet their baseline requirements.

The more active you are, the more calories you need beyond this basic amount. How much more depends on your level of activity. A lumberjack will need more calories than a desk-bound accountant.

Also, the more muscle mass you have the higher your basal metabolic rate is because muscle is metabolically active.

Activity and exercise aren't the only things that require additional calories. Other factors, including stress, injury and wound healing, also increase the need for energy above the baseline requirement.

Actually measuring someone's metabolic rate is quite complicated. It's usually only done for research purposes. However, there are a number of formulas that provide a reasonably accurate rough estimate. These formulas are usually based on factors such as height and weight and age and gender.

The simplest formula is 16 calories per day per pound of lean body mass. Lean body mass does not include fat weight so you need to have at least a general idea of your percent body fat to determine your lean body mass from the weight your scale shows.

For example, if you weigh 150 lbs. and you percent body fat is 20%, then your lean body mass is 120lbs. (150 x .20 = 30 lbs body fat; 150 − 30 = 120 lbs. lean mass)

There are several ways of determining percent body fat. Unfortunately the most accurate methods tend to be the most inconvenient and the least available.

Researchers consider hydrostatic underwater weighing to be the most accurate method. With this method a person's weight on dry ground is compared to their weight underwater. Because body fat and muscle have different densities the amount of change in these two measurements varies according to the percent of body fat. Obviously getting this measurement performed isn't simple.

An instrument called the BodPod is almost as accurate and much more convenient. With this method the person being evaluated sits inside a sealed capsule and the amount of air they displace is measured. This is quicker, easier and more comfortable than underwater weighing. However it's not widely available.

Dual energy X-ray absorptiometry (DEXA) scanning is more widely available. It is based on the fact that tissues of different densities absorb x-rays at a different rate. It is most commonly used to evaluate bone density and people concerned about osteoporosis. However, using different software the same instrument can be used to measure percent body fat as well as bone density. This method of measurement is accurate and consistent. The problem you may run into is finding a scanner set up to measure body fat as well as bone density. In body-conscious California, there's one on every other street corner. In upstate New York, not so much.

Another common method is to use calipers to measure the thickness of subcutaneous fat and then plug these numbers into a formula to estimate percent body fat. The accuracy depends on the formula used and the consistency of taking measurements in the same location. If you're interested in this method you can find calipers and formulas online or get it done at most health clubs.

Bioelectrical impedance is very convenient but can be off by as much as 2 to 4%. This method passes a tiny, undetectable electric current through the body. Because muscle and fat conduct electricity differently variations in body fat shift the impedance measured. In practice, the device is usually incorporated into a scale. You push a button, step on the scale and in a minute have an accurate weight in a pretty good guess at your percent body fat.

While not entirely accurate, this method does give a reasonable estimate and is useful for following trends. It's important to know that your state of hydration significantly influences the results. Most people will get the most consistent results if they measure their percent body fat in the morning before they drink anything.

Before moving on, I want to mention that knowing percent body fat is a very important aspect of a wellness or weight loss program. If someone starts on an exercise program and improves their diet they're likely to lose body fat and gain muscle mass. Losing a pound of fat and gaining a pound of muscle is a tremendous positive change, but seeing the same weight on the scale can be very discouraging. Using the percent body fat to see what's really going on helps avoid this.

Even if you use one of the less accurate methods, such as caliper measurements or bioelectrical impedance they can be quite helpful for following trends. Just be sure to obtain the measurements in a consistent fashion.

By whatever method you attain it, once you know your percent body fat you can use the formula above to calculate your basal metabolic rate.

The more active you are, the more calories you need beyond this basal number. If you're active and trying to heal a wound as well the daily requirement is higher still.

The numbers below are a rough guide as to how energy needs increase with activity. To get an estimate of your calorie needs, multiply your basal metabolic rate by the factor appropriate for your level of activity.

**sedentary** (little or no exercise): multiply BMR x 1.2

**lightly active** (light exercise/sports 1-3 days/week): multiply BMR x 1.375

**moderatetely active** (moderate exercise/sports 3-5 days/week): multiply BMR x 1.55

**very active** (hard exercise/sports 6-7 days a week): multiply BMR x 1.725

**extra active** (very hard exercise/sports & physical job): multiply BMR x 1.9

Here's the main point I want to make here:

Recovering from serious illness can require as many additional calories as being moderately or very active, *even if your physical activity is reduced*.

So that's a rough approximation of an answer to the question "How many calories do you need?" The next question is where should the calories come from?

These calories will come from the three macronutrient categories: carbohydrates, proteins and fats. Carbohydrates and proteins each provide about 4 calories per gram (there are about 28 g in an ounce) while fat provides 9. Considerable debate surrounds the question of what percentage of your daily calories should come from each category.

Let's start with the USDA guidelines. The average recommendations are 55% calories from carbohydrate, 15% from protein, and 30% from fat.

It's difficult for the government to do anything that people won't argue about and dietary guidelines are no different. Several nutritional experts argue against these overall guidelines and I tend to agree with these experts. I believe, especially for active people and people trying to heal wounds, that a lower percentage of calories from carbohydrates and a higher percentage from protein would be better.

In fairness to the USDA, their recommendations are somewhat more flexible than usually reported. The range of percentage calories they suggest is: carbohydrate: 45–65%, protein: 10–35% and fat: 20–35%.

Consider one alternative recommendation. Dr. Barry Sears ( a biochemist, not a *real* doctor :- ) developed and popularized the Zone Diet. Dr. Sears recommends 40% of calories from carbohydrate, 30% from protein and 30% from fat. As you can see these recommendations aren't necessarily that different from the range of calories in the USDA guidelines.

Some people argue that the percentage of fat allowed in both the USDA guidelines and diets such as the Zone and Atkin's diet is too high. Part of the issue here is that not all fats are equal. Exactly what kind of fat you have in your diet makes a huge difference. We'll be talking about this in more detail soon, but for now realize that there is a big difference between various types of fat.

For example, the fat in grain-fed beef (the kind available in most supermarkets) is unhealthy. In contrast, olive oil in moderation is a healthy addition to a person's diet. And almost all of us would benefit from having more fish oil in our diet.

Other people argue against higher percentages of protein. One claim is that increasing protein automatically means a higher percentage of unhealthy fat as well. Another worry is that too much protein somehow damages the kidneys. As we'll see, neither claim is necessarily true.

On balance, I'm not sure how precisely you need to measure your percent calories. I personally like healthy fat in the range of 20-30% with plenty of protein. Carbohydrates should be almost exclusively complex, unrefined carbohydrates. This means no sugars or highly refined processed foods. Crackers, pretzels, chips, bagels, snack foods and much more that are standard fare in the typical diet are all in this category.

Going even further, I personally think that most of the carbohydrates in your diet should be from legumes (beans, lentils, etc.), vegetables and fruits and relatively few from grains, even whole grains such as whole wheat bread, brown rice, etc. But that's another issue...

As it stands, almost anything would be an improvement over the typical American diet. According to the National Health and Nutrition Examination Survey (NHANES) done in 2005-2006 the top sources of calories in the average American diet are:

- Cakes, cookies and other such desserts
- Yeast breads
- Chicken
- Soda and soft drinks
- Pizza

That list is pretty scary. Notice the complete absence of any fruits or vegetables. Chicken is about the only potentially healthy food on that list, but I dread to think what proportion of that chicken is fried chicken or fast food "chicken nuggets" (whatever they are).

Bread could have some value but I'm willing to bet that the vast majority of bread in most Americans' diet is highly refined white bread which is devoid of nutrients and has a devastating effect on a person's blood sugar. White bread is another source of empty calories.

I think you can see that there's room for lots of improvement.

Let's look at each macronutrient in more detail, particularly as they affect wound healing. I intend the information that follows to help you make wiser food choices than most people are doing now.

We'll begin with carbohydrates.

# 3 CARB SENSE

Here's a bold claim: carbohydrates are the root cause of the epidemic of obesity and diabetes in this country. This is not because carbohydrates are bad. They aren't. It's because we eat too many of them and even more because we eat the wrong ones.

Grains, legumes, vegetables, and fruits are all carbohydrates. Refined sugars such as table sugar and high fructose corn syrup are also carbohydrates. Regrettably, the latter bunch has become a major source of carbohydrate calories in the modern American diet.

In their whole form, predominately carbohydrate foods（vegetables, beans, etc.）also contain fiber and a slew of other beneficial nutrients, the micronutrients we'll talk about later.

But these aren't the kind of carbohydrates most Americans eat. Most Americans get a huge percentage of their daily calories from sugar in one form or another and white flour. No fiber, no nutrients — they're eating only empty calories.

25

The empty calorie issue is bad enough, but it gets even worse. <u>These types of carbohydrates knock our finely tuned metabolisms completely out of whack</u>.

The type of carbohydrate we ingest profoundly affects our internal hormonal balance. Although we've only paid much attention to this in the last 20 to 30 years, you'll see that it's of critical importance. These hormonal changes are why so many people find it impossible to lose weight and why so many people are now diabetic.

To begin to explain a new way of thinking about carbohydrates, I want to first mention a concept known as the Glycemic Index.

## Glycemic Index

In the past, we didn't distinguish much between the types of carbohydrates the way we do with fats. While we've thought for some time that there were good fats and bad fats, the same wasn't true about carbohydrates. A carbohydrate was a carbohydrate.

It now seems odd that the differentiation of the effects of carbohydrates was so late in coming because we all intuitively sense the principle behind it. We all know that we feel different if we have a donut for breakfast as opposed to having the same number of calories as oatmeal. The ways these two foods affect our blood sugar levels and our hormonal levels are completely different. This is why we feel differently after we eat them.

There is a huge difference between the effects on the body of something that doesn't require any digestion and is absorbed immediately (the donut) and a complex carbohydrate that needs to be broken down and digested before it can be absorbed (the oatmeal).

It's become clear that the metabolic effects of different carbohydrates have health consequences. Researchers have therefore developed different ways of categorizing them.

You most often hear carbohydrates referred to as "complex", meaning they're in a relatively unrefined state, or "simple", meaning they've been processed with a loss of at least some (usually all) of their nutrients. In this context, whole wheat bread is a complex carb while white bread is a simple carb.

While somewhat helpful, this distinction is fairly general. Nutritionists wanted a more precise and comprehensive way of evaluating a carbohydrates affect on our blood sugars and therefore its effect on our hormonal response. The result was the glycemic index.

The glycemic index attempts to quantify how a given carbohydrate affects a person's blood sugar levels. It attempts to quantify the effect of food, especially carbohydrates, on our metabolism.

The way it is usually reported, table sugar is given a glycemic index of 100. If another food also has a glycemic index of 100, that means the food has the same effect on blood glucose levels as table sugar.

If a food has a glycemic index of less than 100 it means that particular food doesn't affect blood sugar as much as table sugar. For example if the food has a glycemic index of 50, it means that eating 100 calories of that food would raise your blood sugar approximately half as high as eating 100 calories of table sugar.

Refined and highly processed foods don't exist in nature. Our bodies are designed and set up to handle foods requiring digestion. High glycemic index foods wreak havoc because they stimulate an extreme response to the extraordinarily high blood sugar levels they cause.

Insulin is a key player in this response.

Insulin, of course, is a crucial hormone. It is primarily responsible for regulation of blood sugar. Most people have heard of it in association with diabetes, but insulin levels play a critical role in our overall health.

As you probably know, insulin is produced by the pancreas. The pancreas releases more insulin when blood sugar levels increase. Insulin speeds up the transport of sugars into cells, which in turn lowers blood glucose levels. The cells use sugars for energy. But there's a limit to how much they need at any given time. Any extra sugar is converted to fat and stored in adipose cells – cells intended for fat storage.

But that's not all insulin does. Not only does insulin promote the formation of storage fat, it also absolutely blocks the mobilization of fat to be used for energy. This means that <u>if insulin levels are high previously stored fat is unavailable to the body to meet its energy needs</u> – <u>*even if blood sugar levels plummet and more energy is needed*</u>.

29

Release of insulin from the pancreas occurs in two stages. Some insulin is "prepackaged" by the pancreas. It is held in what amounts to small containers just inside the cell membrane ready to be released when needed. This is the immediate response insulin.

If additional insulin is required the pancreas produces it from scratch. This takes time and there is some lag before newly produced insulin is released.

This is a nicely tuned system and works well when we're eating real food, but the modern diet throws a monkey wrench into the works.

If you eat something that is highly refined and absorbed immediately (say, you have a glass of orange juice and some jelly on a bagel for breakfast), those carbohydrates shoot the blood sugar sky-high.

The pancreas responds by immediately dumping its stored insulin, and also by ramping up to produce a lot more.

However, there is no "staying power" with that meal. The initial insulin response is more than enough to lower the blood sugar and further production of insulin isn't required.

Meanwhile, the signal has already been sent. The body is responding as if you ate a meal that is still being digested and will require more insulin. The immediate response insulin has been dumped into the bloodstream and the pancreas gears up to produce more.

This longer-term insulin production is slower to turn on and turn off. That means that after a high glycemic index meal blood sugar levels plummet as the pancreas continues to produce and release insulin. This now drives blood sugars too low, and because insulin levels are high fat stores can't be released to meet the energy needs. This causes carbohydrate cravings.

This is why someone who has coffee and a couple doughnuts for breakfast feels hungry again a few hours later. This typically has them looking for another doughnut or a candy bar to feed the craving.

Contrast this to what happens when you eat the same number of calories as oatmeal.

The oatmeal needs to be digested. The carbohydrates it contains can't be absorbed immediately. Digestion takes place slowly, which means the blood sugar level only rises gradually and never get especially high.

As result, the pancreas responds much more moderately. Small amounts of insulin are released steadily as the oatmeal is gradually digested and absorbed. Blood glucose levels stay in a normal range. The whole process takes quite a bit of time and we feel satisfied longer.

This is the reason we say oatmeal "sticks to your ribs."

To use another metaphor, you might compare high glycemic index foods to lighting a pile of crumpled newspaper in a fireplace as opposed to having a fire with a solid log. The newspaper will flare up and burn very hot, but only for a moment. The log takes longer to get going but will provide steady heat for some time.

One of the things that surprised me when I first started learning about glycemic index is that white bread, that staple of the American diet (I cringe to think how many loaves of Wonder Bread I personally consumed as a kid), has the same or even greater effect on blood sugar as pure table sugar. That is, 100 calories of bread can raise your blood sugar as high or higher as eating 100 calories of sugar.

This is because the carbohydrate in white bread is a simple starch. The enzymes in your saliva are enough to break it down into a form ready for immediate absorption.

Part of the point here is that foods don't have to taste sweet or even have sugar in them to have a dramatic effect on your blood glucose.

Another point is that processing a food dramatically influences its glycemic index.

An example is the oatmeal we were just talking about. In general, oatmeal is a healthy, low glycemic index food. However, processing can change that significantly.

Steel cut oatmeal has a very low glycemic index. The grain has simply been chopped. Second lowest is rolled oatmeal. The grain has been steamed slightly and flattened. Quick oatmeal has been partially cooked and dried again. This process starts to break down the cell walls of the oatmeal. This means that when

33

you eat it, the oatmeal will digest more quickly. This raises the glycemic index somewhat, but it's still relatively low

Instant oatmeal (the heat-in-the-microwave and eat kind) is worse. This has been completely cooked, dried and ground fine. This heavy-handed processing "pre-digests" the oatmeal even more raising its glycemic index tremendously. Worse yet, producers usually load this form of oatmeal with sugar (typically the equivalent of 6 teaspoons of table sugar) as well as artificial flavors — chemicals that no one needs.

What started out as a healthy grain has become only moderately better than a candy bar. And the food manufacturers still get to call this "food like substance" oatmeal. Nutritionally, it bears little resemblance to the initial product.

The underlying principle here is that the closer food is to its raw, native state the healthier it is likely to be. Excessive processing and manipulation strips nutrients and, as the oatmeal example shows, changes the way food affects your body's metabolism.

The glycemic index is a useful number to be familiar with. It can be helpful to learn what the glycemic index of various foods are to help you make wise food choices.

However, this is not anything you should obsess about. You certainly don't need to know the glycemic index of everything you eat. As a basic principle, if you eat food close to its natural state and minimally processed you'll be all right.

Also keep in mind that what's important in the real world is the total glycemic index of a meal. This depends on what combination of foods you eat at a given meal. Two foods consistently lower the glycemic index of a meal: fiber and fat.

This is a reason to include at least a little healthy fat with most meals. Not only does fat itself have little effect on blood sugar, it also slows digestion in general.

When you're making food selections, another food rule to keep in mind is "don't eat anything that comes wrapped in cellophane." Food companies rarely make anything healthier when they package it. The vast majority of time they take something that was reasonably healthy and make it less so.

If I had to pick one thing I could change in the American diet it would be to eliminate sugar and its various forms (fructose, corn syrup, etc.) along with refined carbohydrates (white flour being a prime example) from the American diet.

Heck, even just eliminating soda would be a major improvement.

I believe it's hard to overstate the damage that chronically elevated blood sugars wreak on a person's metabolic system. My belief is that this is a major contributor to the epidemic of obesity and type II diabetes in our country today. Type II diabetes used to also be known as adult onset diabetes because it only happened in adults. We can't call it that any longer because so many children are developing it. Poor diet and lack of exercise underlie this tragic epidemic.

Dr. Mehmet Oz uses a metaphor that I think is very effective and disturbingly accurate. He says we should think of excess sugar molecules circulating in the bloodstream as shards of glass. Can you imagine the damage shards of glass would cause circulating through your body?

One reason high sugar levels are a problem is because they are pro-inflammatory. They tend to set off the body's inflammatory response system even when there is no need for it. We are increasingly realizing that this low-grade inflammation underlies many of the chronic health problems that are becoming so common today.

For example, we now recognize that a slight elevation of a marker of inflammation (C. reactive protein) is associated with an increased rate of heart disease. One current theory is that microscopic, inflammatory injury to the lining of blood vessels sets off the process that allows hardening of the arteries to develop. If the vessel walls weren't inflamed to begin with, high cholesterol levels wouldn't lead to plaque (hardening of the arteries) building up on the inside of arteries.

Also, sugar at high levels can form abnormal combinations with various proteins, creating what are called "advanced glycolation end products" (which has a very appropriate acronym: AGE). These proteins don't function normally and are partly responsible for the complications of long-standing diabetes, such as renal failure and blindness.

A marker that reflects the formation of AGE proteins is hemoglobin A-1 C. Hemoglobin A-1 C levels reflect average blood glucose levels over the last 3 to 4 months. A healthy level should be under six. Even better is a level under 5.7.

So, to repeat, "Eat real food, mostly vegetables, not too much." Also keep in mind the suggestions to not eat anything your great grandparents wouldn't recognize as food and think twice before you eat anything that comes wrapped in cellophane. You could do much worse than use these suggestions as your guide to the foods you pick.

Unfortunately, most of the abundance you see in your local grocery store doesn't count as real food.

I mean really... cookies and crackers and snack foods? What about the soda aisle? These foods have plenty of calories but no nutrients. Extreme processing strips any nutrient that might have once been present in the raw ingredients of any snack food. Soda is only flavored sugar water to begin with.

Every grocery store has a whole aisle devoted to cereal. It may as well be another aisle of cookies and crackers. Look at the labels on the packages. Even the one's pretending to be healthy are usually terrible.

Many of them get most of their calories from sugar and the other half from highly refined grains.

Even though you can get a good idea that a cereal isn't anything you want to put in your body from reading the required nutritional label most people still take things at face value. Here's a story to illustrate the point.

Friends of Jackie and mine came with their kids to stay with us for a few days. They knew that our breakfast cereal selection is limited to oatmeal and a very high fiber cereal. They also knew their kids wouldn't touch either one so they brought along a box of their own cereal. (As much as I like to provide for guests, I just couldn't bring myself to buy the Fruit Loops or whatever it was they were eating.)

Come Sunday morning, my friend Mike went out for the newspaper and brought back some donuts as well. I'll admit to a sweet tooth, so I was fine having some donuts around on a Sunday morning. All things in moderation.

As you might expect, the kids wanted to dig into the donuts right away but dad told them they'd have to wait until after they had their breakfast cereal.

I didn't say anything, but the truth of it is that there really wasn't much nutritional difference between the donut and the cereal. Well actually there was, and it was in the donuts' favor – the donuts probably didn't have as much artificial flavoring and preservatives added as the cereal did, not to mention whatever chemicals it took to give the kids' cereal its gaudy color.

The phrase "you are what you eat" is part of the popular culture. Most people attribute it to the British TV show of that name or perhaps Adelle Davis and other organic food advocates of the 60s and 70s.

Its actual origin resides further back in history. Victor Lindlahr published You Are What You Eat – How to Win and Keep Healthy with Diet in 1942. If Mr. Lindlahr was concerned with the state of the nation's diet in 1942 I wonder what he would think today.

The food we eat is the raw material of our bodies. The quality of the raw ingredients definitely affects the condition of our body.

We are fortunate to have access to a wide range of foodstuffs, both good and bad. Obviously it would be wise to choose the good stuff, but we don't have to. We're free to choose the junk.

For millennia the main issue facing humanity was avoiding starvation. Just getting enough calories was an issue. That's still a problem in many parts of the world but certainly not in the United States, even among those living below the poverty level. Poverty used to be indicated by thinness. In the US some of the highest rates of obesity are among the poor.

So again, for most of us the problem isn't getting enough food, it's making poor choices from all the foods available.

Carbohydrates are definitely part of a healthy diet. Slowly digesting (low glycemic index) carbohydrates are a good energy source. Some organs, the brain in particular, function best with the glucose most readily available from carbohydrates.

Unrefined carbohydrates also provide fiber which is important for bowel function, modulates digestion, lowers overall glycemic index and can help improve lipid profiles. Additionally many carbohydrate foods, especially fruits and vegetables, contain a wealth of micro nutrients. There'll be more on that later. For now, let's move on to the next macro nutrient: protein.

41

# 4 PROTEIN ESSENTIALS

Protein is another macro nutrient. The building blocks of proteins are amino acids, which are linked together in various combinations. The body can break down the proteins we eat into their component amino acids and rearrange them into completely new proteins. It's a remarkable biochemical process. These new proteins can be, for example, muscle fibers or enzymes or antibodies.

Not only that, our biochemical mechanisms have the ability to transform one amino acid into another that is needed. However, the chemical factories of our bodies have their limits. There are some amino acids the body can't produce on demand. These amino acids need to be in the diet for optimum health. Because they have to be provided in the diet, they are referred to as essential amino acids.

Amino acids that the body can readily produce from other raw material are nonessential amino acids.

There is a third group of amino acids that the body can produce, but only in limited amounts. Under some conditions, the need outstrips the production capabilities. These amino acids are called conditionally essential. As you'll see, this has implications for wound healing.

It is of note that our bodies have no storage form of protein. All the protein in our body is biologically active. All of it is performing some needed function.

Excess calories, whether from carbohydrate, protein or fats, are stored as body fat. To a limited extent, that fat can be mobilized to be used as energy in the form of fatty acids. But the stored fat cannot be converted back to glucose. This is a problem because some parts of the body (especially the brain) require glucose as their energy source.

Fatty acids and fats can't be converted into glucose but proteins can.

In a starvation state, if the diet doesn't provide enough carbohydrate the body will start breaking down functional protein to meet its glucose needs.

It's like one of those old movies where the homesteaders run out of fuel in the middle of a blizzard and start burning their furniture and parts of their house in an effort to stay warm. They're meeting the emergency need, but at the expense of the overall well being of their home.

This is one reason why extremely low calorie diets are a poor way to lose excess weight. Once you get below 800 or so calories a day about half the weight you lose is coming from protein (for example muscle mass) that you want to keep, not the fat you want to lose.

Successful wound healing requires protein in the diet. Exactly how much depends on the severity of the wound, ongoing protein losses and the persons pre-existing nutritional status. The increased need for protein can vary anywhere from 25% to 100% more protein than a person needs when they aren't trying to heal a wound.

It's best to eat some protein at regular intervals throughout the day. In fact, it's a good idea to have a mix of protein, carbohydrate and fat at every meal.

One of the objections some people raise against recommending increased protein in the diet is that some sources of protein have a lot of unhealthy fat along with the protein. This especially applies to grain fed beef. As a classic example, a hamburger contains a reasonable amount of protein but it also contains a lot of unhealthy saturated fat.

The same could be said of cheeses. We want quality protein without excessive fat. This means you need to look for lean sources of protein or protein with healthy types of fat.

Lean sources of protein include chicken breast without the skin. Most of the fat in chicken and other poultry is in the skin and the leg meat.

Fish is another good protein source. Mild white fish such as tilapia and catfish are low in fat. Other fish, such as salmon, are relatively high in fat, but the fat is healthy fat that most of us need more of – omega-3 fats.

A readily available inexpensive source of quality proteins is eggs. Whole eggs do have a fair amount of fat as well as cholesterol. However, all the fat and cholesterol is in the yolk. Egg whites are pure protein.

I don't worry about one or two egg yolks a day as far as cholesterol goes, especially if someone has normal blood levels of cholesterol. However most of us don't need the extra fat and calories in the egg yolk. The answer is to eat more whites than yolks.

I often have 2-4 egg whites from regular eggs along with one whole egg that's high in omega-3's. The latter is produced by giving chickens feed that contains omega-3 foods such as flax seed. These are a little more expensive, which is why I use regular eggs for their whites. Why pay a premium for a yolk that you're going to throw out?

Beef and red meat in general have a poor reputation as a source of protein because of the fat associated with them. However, this poor reputation has more to do with how we raise beef cattle today, not with something inherent in red meat.

I highly recommend that you find a source for grass fed beef. I'll talk about this more in the section on fats, but the fat content and nutritional profile of cattle that's been raised on a diet of grass is entirely different from that of the typical feedlot, grain-fed animal. It's different enough that there really is no comparison. It's as if they are two different types of food.

Availability of grass fed beef varies significantly around the country, but it's getting easier to find. One of the supermarkets where I live has started carrying a few cuts of grass fed beef. I've also found some local suppliers at regional farmer's markets.

Sources will vary with where you live, but nationwide you can reliably order grass fed beef online. Before I found it locally, I ordered from several different merchants and had a good experience with all of them.

Whether you buy locally or online, you will pay a premium if you compare on price per pound alone.

However a direct, pound for pound price comparison really isn't fair because the quality of the beef is so different. Besides, even if the price differential is twice as much (it usually isn't that high but it can be) I think it is a much wiser decision to eat 4 – 6 ounces of grass fed steak than twice that amount from an animal that's been raised in a feedlot.

Another good source of very lean red meat that tastes similar to beef is bison (buffalo). Almost by definition buffalo is grass fed and free range since these animals have never been domesticated and don't deal well with being corralled. Buffalo tastes much like beef, yet has a much lower fat content. Some supermarkets are beginning to carry it but it's still a little hard to find. Fortunately, like grass fed beef, buffalo is readily available online.

Another objection I sometimes hear to a high protein diet is that it may cause kidney damage. I've been unable to find any study demonstrating this. I think the confusion may arise because it is true that someone with poor kidney function may need to be careful with the amount of protein they eat because their poorly functioning kidneys can't clear the metabolic byproducts of protein metabolism. This does <u>not</u> mean that protein <u>causes</u> kidney damage.

Obviously, someone with kidney problems needs to check with their nephrologist to determine how much protein is safe for them.

In addition to eating whole foods, protein powders can be a helpful source of added protein. I'll discuss this more in the section on supplements. For now, let's move onto what is perhaps the most controversial and maligned of the macronutrients: fats.

# 5 FATS: THE GOOD THE BAD AND THE REALLY UGLY

Ah, fats... Fats have been one of the most controversial components of diet over the last several decades. The debates rage on, but I believe a consensus is emerging. In this section I'll give a little historical background, and then explain things as I see them now.

Several decades ago studies suggested that there was an increased rate of heart disease in many people with a diet high in saturated fats. Nutritionists and doctors responded by labeling all saturated fats as "bad."

Then, as if it wasn't enough to blame fat for heart disease, it became fashionable to blame it for the obesity epidemic as well.

When this happened, low fat diets became the rage.

I wish I could say I recognized the foolishness in all this, but I didn't. The recommendations I made to my patients back then are a source of embarrassment to me now. I suppose it's a good thing that most of them ignored me anyway.

51

In the 1980s I enthusiastically recommended an extremely low fat vegetarian diet program to my patients with vascular disease. At the time, it wasn't an unreasonable thing to do. Dr. Ornish actually had studies showing reversal of vascular disease (heart disease in particular) in people who adhered to his program. If you're interested, you can read about it in <u>Dr. Dean Ornish's Program for Reversing Heart Disease</u>.

There were two problems with my recommending the diet. The first is that the positive results Dr. Ornish reported came from a complete program, not just the diet. The program included smoking cessation, moderate exercise, yoga, meditation, and group support as well as the diet.

It was a complete package that yielded the great results, yet people focused mainly on the diet.

A second problem is that the diet Dr. Ornish recommends is just about impossible for most of us to stay with. It's completely vegetarian with less than 10% of calories coming from any form of fat and zero dietary cholesterol.

I think you'll agree that's a little restrictive.

I'm usually pretty good at staying with something I think is healthy, but even I had trouble staying with that. My vegetarian phase on the Ornish plan only lasted a couple of years. I don't think any of the hundreds of patients I recommended it to stuck with it either.

As an aside, during my vegetarian phase I lost a lot of muscle mass.

These days, I think there's another problem with diets that focus solely on avoiding fat. Today, it's possible to follow Dr. Ornish's dietary fat and cholesterol guidelines and still eat an extremely unhealthy diet. This is because of the food industries response to the low-fat craze.

When Dr.Ornish outlined his original diet, non-fat package goods didn't exist. If you ate a cookie or cracker, it had fat in it. This meant that if you followed the Ornish diet when it first came out you automatically were eating unprocessed foods and lots of vegetables, fruits and whole grains.

That sounds a lot like the diet we've been talking about, minus the meat and healthy fat.

The food industry responded to the interest in low-fat foods by producing – Ta Daaaa.... low-fat everything. Low fat and nonfat cakes, cookies and ice cream filled supermarket shelves. These foods remained devoid of any nutrients, were high in sugar and

53

refined, high glycemic index grains, and had the added bonus of nonfood chemicals added to make up for the taste, texture and "mouth feel" of the missing fats.

This was not a healthy turn of events. The resulting products are not nutritious food. Rather they are another example of food like substances. The products have a high glycemic index (not good), are nutrient poor, and contain a host of chemicals we just don't need.

As you can see, once again the advice to "eat real food, mostly vegetables, not too much" proves itself to be useful. Most processed and packaged foods just aren't good for us.

As far as I know, Dr. Ornish still recommends his program with the proviso of staying with whole foods and avoiding processed foods, even non-fat ones. That might be a healthy diet for some folks but I don't think it's the best for the vast majority of people.

Following the low-fat/high carb fad, the dietary fashion pendulum swung in the opposite direction giving rise to high protein/high fat low carb diets. The Atkins diet typified this trend.

In general I think this approach is an improvement but I <u>don't</u> think the Atkins Diet specifically is the way to go. This is primarily because Dr. Atkins completely ignored both the amount and the type of fats he recommended. If you're interested in one of these dietary models I think the South Beach Diet is more prudent.

All of this seems to be the classic medical muddle where what was supposedly bad for you yesterday is now good for you and visa versa and no one knows what to believe. While I'll admit it does seem that way, I think there are some sensible principles arising. I'll lay them out for you here as best I can.

For one thing, I think it's best to include at least a moderate amount of fat in the diet. This does not mean we can consume an endless amount of fat (a la Atkins). We also need to pay attention to the type of fats we consume.

When thinking about fats, keep the following points in mind.

All fats are calorie dense. That is, they have a lot of calories in a small volume. It's easy to eat more calories than you need without realizing it. A good example of this is nuts. While 20 or so almonds a day might be a healthy addition to your diet, I find it easy to eat nuts by the handful. Going overboard adds more fat and calories than I need.

The fact is proteins and carbohydrates each provide about 4 calories per gram. Fat has nine or 10. If you eat a lot of fat, you will probably take in more calories than you need unless you're working as a lumberjack.

You also need to know that not all fats act the same way in our bodies. Different categories of fats have different effects on our metabolism. We know enough about these effects to make reasonable decisions concerning the fats in our diet.

To give you the summary first, we should:

- increase the amount of omega-3 fats in our diet
- reduce the amount of saturated fats
- completely avoid trans fats
- use mono-unsaturated fats (or I could just say use olive oil) in our cooking and
- get most vegetable oils (safflower oil, corn oil, etc.) out of the kitchen.

An addendum might be to use some coconut oil and eat a few nuts.

Here's what I mean by all that.

I'll begin with a little chemistry about fats. You really don't need to know this stuff so feel free to ignore it and skip ahead if you like. Making healthy food choices doesn't require knowing chemistry.

But if you are interested in a bit of the chemistry, here it is.

Fats are made up of molecules called fatty acids. Fatty acids are carboxylic acid molecules with chains of carbon attached.

These carbon atoms can have different types of connections between them and they also can connect with various numbers of hydrogen atoms.

One way chemists classify fatty acids is according the number of carbon atoms they have, the type and location of the connections between these carbon atoms and how many hydrogen molecules are attached.

Based on the location of the first carbon double bond in the molecule, fatty acids are classified as omega-3, omega-6 and omega-9.

As we've already seen, the human body is an amazing chemical plant. It produces an astounding

57

numbers of compounds on demand using remarkably flexible cellular chemistry to do so.

However, the human biochemical factory has its limits. It can't produce everything from any raw material. Some specific raw materials need to be provided in the diet. If the diet is deficient, the body has to make do with what it has. This is not good for health.

This applies to some fatty acids. There are many fatty acids the body can produce as needed, but there are some it can't. These fatty acids need to be in the diet. Because of this, we call them essential fatty acids. The concept is very similar to the idea of essential amino acids which we talked about earlier.

That's a long explanation to get to this point. Omega 9 fatty acids are not essential so you don't need to worry about trying to specifically include them in your diet.

Some omega 3 and omega 6 fatty acids are essential fatty acids. If they're not in your diet, your body has to make do with other fatty acids.

But (as they say on the infomercials) there's more...

As important as it is to have both kinds of essential fatty acids in your diet, it's also important to have the right ratio of fatty acids. That is, the right balance between omega 3 and omega 6 fatty acids.

This is another area where most people go wrong.

The typical American diet contains way too much omega 6 fat and not enough omega 3s. Omega 3 and omega 6 fatty acids both use the same enzyme process to be converted to other chemicals the body needs. If there's too much omega 6 around, it's going to crowd out the omega 3 fatty acids, even if they're present in reasonable amounts.

Nutritionists estimate that the ideal ratio for health is 1:2 to 1:5 of omega 3 to omega 6 fatty acids.

Today's diet has a ratio of 1:20 or even higher!

High ratios contribute to over activation of the inflammatory system, poor immune response, vascular disease and even cancer.

On the other hand, a low ratio supports health. As an example, a diet with an omega 3 to omega 6 ratio of 1:4 is associated with a 70% reduction in the risk of heart disease.

So here's the deal: the typical American diet has too much fat overall, with mainly unhealthy fats and not enough of omega 3 fatty acids and other healthy fats. We pay the price for it with our health.

We'll talk about this more in a little while. Specifically, I'll make some suggestions to help you get a more healthy balance of fats in your diet. But first I want to explain another way of categorizing fats.

## Saturated Fats, Unsaturated Fats, Mono Unsaturated Fats and Trans Fats

When describing fats, the term "saturated" refers to how many hydrogen ions are present in the fat molecule. If it's holding the maximum amount that's possible chemically, we call it saturated. If there's room for more hydrogen ions, it's unsaturated. If there's only room for one more hydrogen atom, it's monounsaturated.

We've known for a long time that a diet high in saturated fats, typically animal fats, is associated with unhealthy blood lipid profiles and an increase risk of heart attacks and vascular disease. That still holds true, which is why we should include only a moderate amount of most saturated fats in our diets. There is an important exception to this rule I'll mention in a moment.

A quick way to know whether a fat is saturated or not is to remember that saturated fats tend to be solid at room temperature. Think of butter and lard.

Unsaturated fats are usually liquid at room temperature. Think corn oil and safflower oil.

Saturated fats are unhealthy, but there's a category of fat that's even worse. These are the trans-fats that you may have heard about. This is another story of food processing taking something that was at least not particularly dangerous and making it extremely unhealthy.

Trans-fats came into being when food manufacturers realized it's possible to chemically modify an unsaturated fat by tweaking it and adding a few hydrogen ions to make it solid at room temperature. The resultant fat of this chemical manipulation is a trans-fat. You see it identified on food labels as a "partially hydrogenated oil."

So when saturated fats moved onto the list of bad fats to be avoided, food manufacturers moved in with their vegetable oil margarine – a product made with partially hydrogenated vegetable oil. When people switched from butter to margarine they were essentially switching from one not so healthy fat to an even more unhealthy fat.

Unfortunately, I not only ate margarine for years myself, I recommended it to patients, buying into the belief that it was an improvement over butter.

As it turns out, trans-fats are probably the least healthy type of fat you can eat. Sometimes after I read papers reporting the effects of trans fats I think any product that contains them ought to have a skull and cross bone on the package.

The good news in all this is I've gone back to eating butter with a clean conscience (just not too much).

Vegetable oils commonly used for cooking (corn oil, safflower oil, etc.) are unsaturated and in the category of omega 6 fats.

In and of themselves, these fats are relatively neutral. They are calorie dense so eating too much can easily contribute to weight gain but they aren't associated with the deleterious effect of saturated fats and trans fats.

However, as I mentioned a little while ago, the ratio of omega-3 fats to omega 6 fats is important because of shared metabolic pathways. Most Americans consume way too much omega-6 and not enough omega-3. To get the ratio of omega-3 to omega-6 down from the typical 1 to 20 to a healthier 1 to 4 most of us will need to eat more omega-3 fats and reduce the amount of omega 6 fats in our diet.

For this reason, I recommend getting vegetable oils (corn oil, safflower oil etc.) out of your kitchen. Instead, use another healthy fat: olive oil. Olive oil is unique for several reasons.

Olive oil is mono unsaturated and is a very traditional cooking oil. People are looking at it in a new light because researchers who study the prevalence of diseases in different countries noticed some time ago that the rate of heart disease was much lower in some European countries despite the fact that they had a higher rate of some risk factors, such as smoking, compared to the US. They noticed that many of the countries with the lower rates of disease bordered on the Mediterranean.

Of course when these types of differences come up it's often very difficult to identify for sure just what the reason is. Perhaps genetic differences are involved. Maybe the lifestyle and close knit community support makes the difference. Such factors certainly are important but there is a growing body of evidence that the diet in these cultures plays a prominent role in the lower disease rates. Olive oil is part of the reason why the so-called Mediterranean diet is so healthy.

For example, a study in Greece (CARDIO2000 case-control study, published in Clinical Cardiology Kontogianni MD, Panagiotakos DB, et al.). looked at olive oil consumption as well as risk factors for cardiac disease. All other things being equal, using olive oil exclusively reduced the occurrence of heart disease by 47%.

Other studies have demonstrated that olive oil lowers both total cholesterol levels and the LDL (bad) form of cholesterol.

Not only that, but olive oil makes the LDL cholesterol that is present more resistant to damage from free radicals, byproducts of metabolism that are highly reactive. This appears to be due to oleic acid (a fatty acid in olive oil). If oleic acid intake is high, it becomes a dominant fatty acid in cholesterol. This version of cholesterol resists oxidation by free radicals. This is important because it is the oxidized form of cholesterol that clings to the lining of blood vessels setting off the cascade of events that lead to hardening of the arteries.

Olive oil also contains a number of other phytonutrients that provide additional health benefits. All of these are most available if the olive oil isn't heated.

Olive oil isn't the only reason the Mediterranean diet protects a person's health.

The Mediterranean diet emphasizes fresh produce, whole grains, beans, nuts and legumes. Traditionally, people shop at the local market every day buying mainly what's in season.

The main source of protein in the Mediterranean diet is fish and seafood. People in these countries consume chicken and other poultry in very moderate amounts and red meat even less so.

Dairy is not very prominent and it's usually consumed in the form of yogurt and cheese.

Refined and processed foods are minimal or absent altogether.

I think you can see that the traditional Mediterranean diet is quite consistent with Pollan's advice to eat food, mostly plants, not too much. I believe some underlying principles are beginning to emerge.

As an aside, more recent studies show that the diet in countries where the Mediterranean diet was first identified has shifted in the last generation or so. It now includes more meat and processed food. As this shift has occurred, disease rates have increased in parallel.

Here's a review of what we've covered so far on fats. We've accepted that we need some fats in our diet, maybe up to 20 or even 30% of calories. We also realize that the types of fat we eat are important. We know to minimize saturated fats and avoid trans fats completely. Vegetable oils are out of the kitchen and olive oil and coconut oil are in.

Let's talk a little more about saturated fats. This primarily means animal fats from meat and dairy products.

Although I don't like processed foods, it really doesn't take much processing to make low fat or non fat milk. In fact, in the days before whole milk was routinely homogenized making skim milk was something you could do at home. If milk isn't homogenized, the fat rises to the top as cream since oil and water don't mix. All you had to do to make skim milk is pour off the cream.

You can't do it at home anymore, but do choose skim milk, non-fat yogurt and low fat cheese. Non-fat cheese generally strikes me as skating too close to the realm of food-like substances, so I generally avoid it.

Remember when I mentioned that the 13% of milk that isn't water is roughly equal parts protein, lactose and fat? That means that whole milk is about 4% fat, which in turn means 2% milk still has a lot of fat. Choose 1% or skim.

Now let's deal with another major source of saturated fat – beef. I want to continue the discussion we started when we were talking about protein.

Most meat sold in this country comes from cattle fed in feed lots.

Cattle in feed lots have an interesting diet. It often includes leftovers and trimmings from food factories. It can include cast-offs, waste or seconds from potato product plants, bakeries, pasta producers and even candy makers.

I don't know of a study to prove it, but somehow I suspect that a diet with a lot of starch and candy in it isn't particularly healthy for a cow.

It certainly isn't natural.

Cattle's natural diet is grass. They can get by on a less than ideal diet, the same way humans do, but it definitely has an affect on their well being.

From our viewpoint, the feed lot diet drastically alters the nutritional profile of the meat. Overall fat content increases dramatically. It's kind of like the way our fat content increases dramatically on a diet of sugars and starches without a lot of activity.

This chart shows the difference in fat content between feedlot beef and other meats:

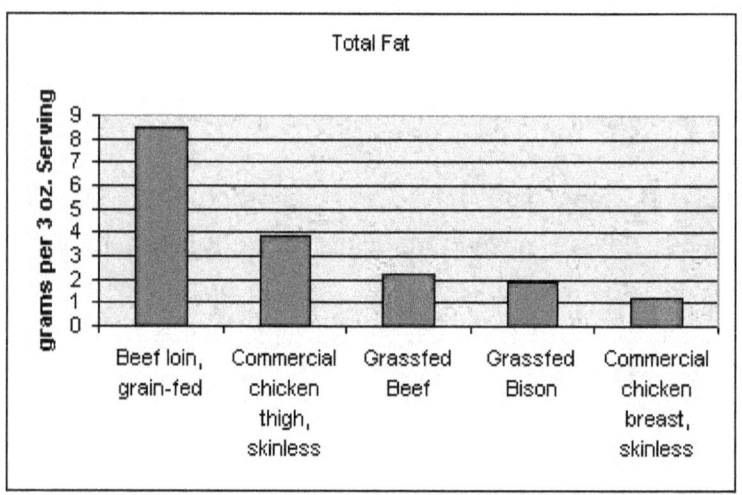

As you can see in that chart, grain-fed beef has more than 4 times as much fat as grass-fed. Grass fed beef is almost as low in fat as skinless chicken breasts.

Not only does the total amount of fat increase when cattle eat grain (and candy byproducts), the kinds of fat in the meat change as well. Grass fed beef contains a healthy portion of omega 3 fats. Meat from grain fed cattle is almost devoid of omega-3 fats. Here's a chart that shows what happens to omega-3 fats in animals raised in a feedlot:

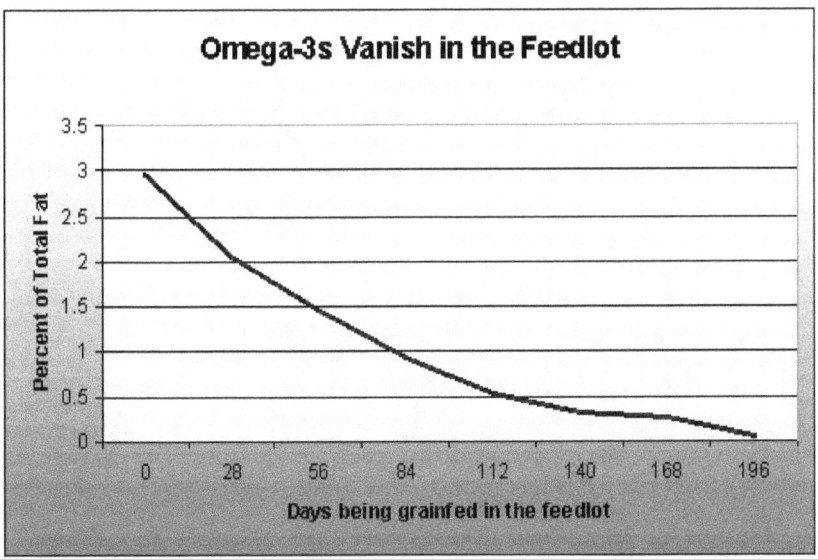

**Omega-3s Vanish in the Feedlot**

Reference: J Animal Sci (1993) 71(8):2079-88

As that chart shows, omega 3s vanish in the feedlot

Grain fed animals have a higher percentage of fat in the meat and this increased fat is unhealthy, with virtually no omega-3 fats.

I think you can see from these charts that the nutritional profile between feed lot beef and grass fed beef is so different that they're almost different foods. I highly recommend you find a source of grass-fed beef or bison.

One point: because grass fed is so lean, the steaks aren't as tender as grain fed. The "marbling" that some people look for as a sign of quality of a steak is actually just the fat induced in the feedlot. That doesn't strike me as a desirable feature.

You can grill grass fed beef, but they do overcook easily. You need to be careful. On the other hand, grass fed beef works extremely well in recipes that call for cooking the meat with moisture, such as chili, stew or pot roast.

## Omega 3 Fat

I've been talking about increasing the omega-3 fats in your diet. Just how do you do that? Well, as we've just seen, one way is to switch to grass fed beef. But it would be better to do even more.

As you probably know, fish oil is high in omega-3 fatty acids. The American Heart Association recommends having at least 2 servings of fish per week.

While including fish in your diet is a good idea, some people don't care for fish. And unfortunately, we all need to be concerned about contaminants such as mercury and PCBs in fish.

For example, I really enjoy tuna, both fresh and canned, but most tuna is contaminated with mercury. With canned tuna I prefer albacore to light, but albacore is higher in mercury so I've switched to light.

As a rough rule, you shouldn't eat more than one can of tuna in a week. Any more and you will begin to accumulate mercury.

I do like to get most of my nutrients from food, but it's prudent to be cautious with seafood consumption. Some fish are especially problematic because they're long-lived and/or high on the food chain. This means they tend to concentrate contaminates over their lifetime. Such fish include swordfish, mackerel, and tilefish. It's best to avoid these.

On a positive note, salmon has low levels of mercury and is also high in omega 3's.

For most of us, I believe it will be difficult to get a healthy amount of omega-3 fats in our diet from food alone.

Personally, I usually have salmon once or twice a week and supplement that dietary intake with fish oil capsules.

Are fish oil capsules free of mercury? Some producers of supplements claim that their product is free of contaminants but others aren't. However, I think that is mainly a marketing ploy. One study in 1998 found detectable levels of contaminants in several brands of supplements, but subsequent studies, including a

71

review by Consumer Reports, show little if any risk with fish oil supplements.

One source of omega-3 fats that I think is probably best avoided is cod liver oil. Although rich in omega-3's it also contains quite a bit of vitamin A which is problematic in large doses. Plus it tastes terrible.

Omega 3's aren't only available in fish. Several plants contain them as well. The most concentrated plant source is flax seed. Two tablespoons contain about 3 1/2 g.

You can buy flax seed oil or capsules, but I recommend that you use the whole seed and grind it just before you use it for a couple of reasons.

Flax is a good source of fiber (5 grams in 2 tbsp) and contains a group of compounds called ligands which have a host of beneficial effects of their own, including suppressing several types of cancer (breast and prostate in particular). They also balance female hormone levels in women.

Another reason to use whole seed and grind it just before you use it is that flax seed oil spoils very easily. You're most assured of getting the full benefits if you grind it yourself.

Flax seed is easy to grind with a coffee mill. Then you can add it to oatmeal or another cereal, blend into yogurt or a smoothie or use it in a salad.

I recommend buying a grinder to use just for flax seed. I tried using our coffee grinder, but it was harder than I thought to get all the coffee out of the grinder. I rapidly discovered that I didn't care for raw coffee grounds on my morning cereal.

You can buy already ground flax seed (flax seed meal); however, it's more expensive than whole seed and needs to be stored carefully. If you buy it, look for a product in an opaque, vacuum sealed package, keep it in the refrigerator and use it within a few weeks of opening.

Walnuts are another reasonable source of omega 3. An ounce of walnuts (about 14 walnut halves) has over two grams.

You should be aware that there are three main omega 3 fatty acids that we need: alpha-linolenic acid (ALA), eicosapentaenoic acid (EPA) and docosahexaenoic acid (DHA). ALA is more prominent in flaxseed oil while fish oils contain more EPA and DHA

The body can convert alpha-linolenic acid to EPA and DHA but isn't always very efficient at it. It's probably

73

best to have all three in your diet and not rely solely on flax seed or flaxseed oil.

Most fish oil capsules contain 1000 mg (1 g) of total oil. The amount of EPA and DHA varies between brands and it is usually listed on the label. One brand I've used recently had 250mg DHA and EPA per capsule while another had 320 mg.

I usually aim for a total of at least 1000 mg of DHA and EPA every day, which works out to 3 or 4 capsules per day. This is a relatively modest amount, but I believe it is enough to make a difference. Some studies use much higher doses – 8, 10 or even 12 g of fish oil per day without significant side effects.

One theoretical concern is that high doses of omega-3 might interfere with blood clotting, especially in someone on blood thinners such as Coumadin or warfarin.

This usually isn't a problem but anyone taking anticoagulants should check with their doctor before taking large doses of fish oil. The main thing will be to take a consistent dose. This will allow your physician to reliably adjust the dose of blood thinner based on lab results.

Another issue that comes up is that some people experience a "fishy" after taste or mild indigestion when they take fish oil. Taking the capsules with meals usually eliminates this problem. Sometimes changing brands will make a difference as well.

If after taste is still a problem, try keeping your fish oil capsules in the freezer.

Another thing to try is to take a digestive enzyme capsule with your meals and fish oil. If the fishy taste or indigestion goes away, it suggests that you may not be producing enough digestive enzymes on your own. In that situation, you should probably take a digestive enzyme regularly to be sure you're able to absorb the nutrients you're eating.

In summary, to add omega 3 fats to your diet, I recommend eating fish (salmon preferred) once or twice a week, supplementing with one or two capsules of fish oil with breakfast and dinner daily and eating 2 tablespoons of ground flax seed daily.

Here's a summary of my overall advice concerning fats:

* Aim for 20-30% of calories from fat.

* Have a small amount of healthy fat with every meal.

* Use olive oil as the predominant oil in your kitchen.

* Completely avoid trans fats.

* Try to include fish in your diet once or twice a week.

* Supplement with fish oil capsules.

* Have 2 tablespoons of freshly ground flaxseed every day.

* Consider using grass fed beef or bison as protein sources.

In addition to these changes, you may also want to consider using coconut oil, both in cooking and as a skin lotion. I didn't want to complicate this chapter by going into this in detail here, but I have written a special report just on coconut oil (I think it's that important). The use of coconut oil is one of those areas where I've changed my mind dramatically in recent years. You can get the report and find out why (for free) by visiting my website at: http://www.jfmccaffreymd.com/coconut-oil.html

We've now discussed carbohydrates, proteins and fats – the three macronutrients. Now it's time to consider micronutrients.

# 6 NUTRIENT DETAILS

Protein, fat and carbohydrate are the big categories. But we need much more to really thrive. We do best with a wide array of micronutrients.

Of course you know about vitamins and minerals, but micronutrients go way beyond these compounds. Unprocessed foods contain an astounding number of chemical elements, many of which significantly affect our health.

When it comes to micronutrients, the emphasis is on fruits and vegetables. While there certainly are micronutrients in protein sources, the widest variety comes from plants.

You may have heard the recommendation to "strive for 5", meaning 5 servings of fruits and vegetables. That's a good start. I'm going to suggest that aiming for 9 servings or more is even better.

## Vegetables

You can't go wrong eating almost any vegetable. I have a few nutritional favorites that I think you should emphasize and eat regularly, but the most important thing is to eat a variety.

Let color be your guide. We refer to the healthy compounds in vegetables as phytonutrients. These nutrients affect the color of a vegetable, so eating a lot of different color vegetables means you're giving your body a wide variety of nutrients to work with.

This makes sense. It's not hard to imagine that you'll get a wider variety of nutrients if you eat carrots, onions, red peppers, winter squash and green beans then if you eat only green beans.

## Fresh vs. Frozen

Many people think that fresh vegetables are nutritionally superior to frozen or canned vegetables. Actually, it depends.

The high temperatures required for canning can indeed reduce the nutrients in many vegetables (although canned spinach works great for Popeye). However these high temperatures are not as much a concern for things such as tomato products or beans and legumes.

The other option is frozen vegetables. These can be nutritionally superior to fresh. Freezing preserves nutrients very well and today's producers usually freeze vegetables within a day, often within hours, of harvest.

If I buy fresh-picked broccoli from a farm stand and have it for dinner that night, that's great.

On the other hand, if I buy broccoli that took a day or two to get to the store, sat in the produce section for another day or two, and then spends four days in the veggie drawer of my refrigerator before I get around to cooking it, I would probably get more nutrition from frozen broccoli.

## Organic vs. Non-Organic

Ideally, we would just get the nutrients in our food without any added chemicals. Specifically, our food would be without any pesticides or herbicides.

While purely organic food is a nice idea, I'm not certain that it would be appropriate to eliminate the use of chemicals from agriculture completely. Let's sidestep that somewhat philosophical discussion and focus on practicalities here.

The fact is that organic produce isn't always available, and when it is you pay a premium.

We also need to keep in mind that some foods are extremely low in pesticide residuals even when raised by non-organic farmers.

I think it's useful to be aware of which foods tend to have high chemical residuals and buy organic versions of these when available.

We can be less careful about foods that can have low residuals.

The foods that most often have high levels of residual chemicals include: strawberries, peaches, apples, pears, bell peppers, cherries, potatoes, spinach, celery and grapes.

If you are unable to buy organic versions of these foods, the next best thing is to wash them well. Most supermarkets carry sprays in the vegetable section that claim to significantly reduce chemical residuals. I haven't seen any studies proving this but I suspect they help to a certain extent.

You can also use a teaspoon or so of dishwashing liquid to a gallon of water. Either way be sure to rinse well.

The list of vegetables that are less likely to carry significant residuals includes: blueberries, broccoli, cabbage, bananas, peas, asparagus, corn, winter squash, avocado and onion. It's probably okay to save some money and buy conventionally raised versions of these foods.

Just about any vegetable is a good vegetable, but some contain such potent phytonutrients that you should make a point to eat them regularly. I'll mention a few of these in a moment.

One point I want to make clear is that although I may highlight one specific nutrient or another as I discuss the vegetables below, I do not mean to imply that these nutrients are the only important compounds in the food nor that taking an isolated supplement of a nutrient can replace eating your veggies.

I believe supplements can help, but they're supplements, not a replacement for real food,

The following are foods to consider regularly including in your diet.

## Garlic

Garlic is high on anyone's list of helpful nutrients. Garlic lowers cholesterol, lowers blood pressure, has anti-inflammatory properties and seems to reduce the incidence of virtually all forms of cancer. There is also some suggestion that it has antiviral and antibacterial properties and supports immune function.

81

All this is in addition to its usefulness in warding off vampires.

Purists insist you should eat your garlic raw but that's little difficult for most of us. Some of the compounds in garlic only reach their active form after enzymes act on them. For example, allin needs to be converted to the active compound allicin. The necessary enzymes to do this are in garlic. These enzymes are activated by chopping the garlic, but they are destroyed by cooking. However if you chop garlic and let it sit for five minutes before cooking the enzymes have a chance to work and allicin is produced.

When I'm cooking a recipe that contains both onions and garlic, as many do, I'll chop the garlic first then let it sit while I chop the onion, let it sit for a while and begin to sauté it. By the time I add the garlic just at the end of cooking, it's had a chance to sit long enough to allow the allicin to develop. In fact, onions have similar benefits and it's a good idea to let them sit for a while after chopping as well.

## Cruciferous vegetables

This is a family of vegetables that includes broccoli, cauliflower and cabbage. While it also includes brussel sprouts, I can't quite bring myself to recommend brussel sprouts since they remain one my least favorite vegetables (apologies to my friend Lynn, who loves them). I keep trying them every now and again, but so far I haven't found a way to prepare them that I enjoy.

Fortunately, I like cabbage a lot and don't mind broccoli and cauliflower.

The reason this class of vegetables is high on my list is because they contain phytonutrients of the class of glucosinolates. These compounds as well as some of their metabolites, including indole 3 carbinol, reduce the incidence of cancer, especially breast, prostate and colon cancer. Obviously, these are very common cancers and anything we can do to reduce their incidence has huge implications.

The beneficial effect of cruciferous vegetables is rather pronounced, leading to exciting research. In fact, researchers at Johns Hopkins have developed and patented a way of producing broccoli sprouts that are particularly high in these compounds. The sprouts are marketed under the name Broccosprouts. A portion of the profits goes to support further research.

In addition these vegetables are a good source of fiber, have mild anti-inflammatory affects and help clear toxins from the body.

Cooking tends to destroy their nutrients. Just how much depends on the method. For example, boiling

83

vegetables in water leeches nutrients from them as they cook. That's why the cooking water becomes discolored. You wind up pouring those nutrients down the drain.

Steaming causes much less disruption, but still reduces the nutrient content somewhat.

I'm not a complete raw food advocate, but fresh, raw vegetables do have the highest nutrient content available. I think it's a good idea to include some raw vegetables in your diet. When you do cook vegetables, avoid over-cooking them.

There are many ways to enjoy these vegetables. Of course, it's easy to steam broccoli and cauliflower, but don't stop there. I'm especially fond of a raw broccoli salad that Jackie makes.

One recipe we picked up from The South Beach Cookbook is to steam cauliflower and then mash it with some low-fat milk and a little butter. Serve it as you would mash potatoes.

Coleslaw is a great way to regularly include cabbage in your diet. The fact that coleslaw is eaten raw is a bonus. There are lots of different recipes for making coleslaw. Jackie is a pro at it and one version or another is probably the most common salad that we have in our home.

# Blueberries

Blueberries are one of the best sources of antioxidants. In addition they are a good source of fiber and also have a relatively low glycemic index. Plus they taste good (a lot better than brussel sprouts).

I buy fresh when they're in season, but most of the year I keep a bag of frozen berries in the freezer.

## Tomatoes and Tomato Products

Have you noticed how the recommendations are changing colors, from white to green to blue to red? A variety of colors indicates a variety of nutrients and potential health benefits.

Tomatoes are high in lycopenes. Lycopenes are good for both men and women, but they're especially important for men. Well-conducted studies show that men who have at least three servings of tomato products a week have a 50% lower rate of prostate cancer. Considering the high rate of prostate cancer, this is a dramatic finding.

Even more impressive, a study in men with dysplasia (pre-cancer) of the prostate found on biopsy showed that men who supplemented with lycopene had a lower rate of prostate cancer and in fact had improved

85

biopsies when they were repeated after six months compared to men who received placebo.

Lycopene is one nutrient whose absorption is actually improved by cooking. You don't need to give up raw tomatoes on your sandwiches or in your salads, but be sure to have some canned salsa or cooked tomato sauce as well.

Of course, tomato sauce gives you another opportunity to add garlic to your diet.

For me, the easiest way to regularly include tomatoes in my diet is to have a glass of low-sodium tomato juice or V-8 juice every morning. It tastes pretty good as is but I like to spice it up some. I add New Salt (New Salt is a brand name for a salt replacement. It contains potassium chloride instead of sodium chloride. You'll probably find it in the salt section at your supermarket), horseradish and hot pepper sauce as well as black pepper.

Tomato juice is naturally high in potassium. Adding New Salt raises the content even more. This is good because most of us can use some extra potassium in our diet. Reducing sodium intake while increasing potassium intake lowers blood pressure much more effectively than just reducing sodium alone.

However, do be careful adding potassium chloride to your diet. Too much can be toxic. If you have children in your home, keep the New Salt away from them.

Also, people with kidney problems have trouble managing potassium. <u>Anyone with any degree of renal failure or other kidney problems definitely needs to check with a doctor before adding potassium to their diet</u>.

## Flaxseed

Flaxseed is one of the best plant sources of omega-3 fats. I spent quite a bit of time in the oil section talking about the importance of including a proper balance of healthy fats in your diet. In particular, I explained how almost all Americans would benefit from increasing their intake of omega-3 oils. That alone makes adding flax seed to your diet a good idea.

But that's only the beginning. Nutrients in flaxseed exert anti-inflammatory effects, help bone strength, protect against cancer, lower cholesterol, lower blood pressure and modulate hormone levels in women, among other good things.

Can you see why I recommend adding flax to your diet? Let's get into some details.

Flaxseeds are the seeds of the flax plant, the plant from which linen fibers are derived. These seeds are small (slightly larger than a sesame seed) and vary in color from tan to reddish brown to dark brown.

Flaxseed contains alpha linolenic acid (ALA), a precursor of EPA and DHA which are the omega-3 fats in fish oil. In addition, flaxseed is high in fiber as well as a group of compounds known as ligands. I'll explain why these ligands are very important in a moment. First let's talk about the effect of flax seed on your body's inflammatory response.

Our bodies are in constant state of flux as they adjust to conditions and circumstances. The balance needs to be just right. The fancy medical name for this is homeostasis.

For example, we don't want our immune system suppressed or we'll find ourselves susceptible to all sorts of infections (think of AIDS as an extreme example). On the other hand, we don't want our immune systems reacting willy-nilly to everything, or we'll have troubles with auto immune diseases, diseases in which the bodies own immune system attacks itself. Rheumatoid arthritis is an example of this.

Similarly, we need a balance in the inflammatory response: not too much, not too little. Part of the reason we need the proper ratio between omega 3 fats and omega 6 fats is that omega-3 fats weigh in on the anti inflammatory side of the scale while omega-6 fats settle on the pro inflammatory side of things. The high ratio of omega-6 to omega-3 fats in the American diet means that most Americans have a mild chronic elevation of inflammatory factors circulating throughout their body.

Flaxseed helps you attain a healthy balance, thereby helping such problems as asthma, arthritis, heart disease and other diseases that have an inflammatory component.

Flaxseed also helps with lipid balance. I don't need to tell you that a lot of people have unhealthy levels of cholesterol. Flax seed improves a person's lipid profile. For example, a small study (40 patients) showed that 20 g of ground flaxseed (about 2 tbsp.) was as effective as statin drugs in lowering cholesterol, only without the risk of side effects associated with statins. Flaxseed probably exerts this effect through a combination of its fiber and omega 3 content.

Now let's get back to the ligands that I mentioned before.

One of the main reasons I recommend whole flax seed over flaxseed oil is the much higher concentration of ligands in whole flaxseed. Even so-called high ligand oil has very little compared to the whole seed.

These compounds are important because they have a powerful affect against two of the most common cancers: breast cancer and prostate cancer. Researchers suspect two mechanisms are at work here.

The first is that ligands block the growth of new blood vessels to the tumor, thereby starving it. (Journal of Clinical Oncology, 2007 ASCO Annual Meeting, Abstract 1510)

The second is that they modulate estrogen metabolism, an important factor in both breast and prostate cancer.

As an aside, for years many people thought that testosterone caused prostate cancer. This turns out to be the medical equivalent of an old wives tale. While it is true that once a man has prostate cancer testosterone might accelerate its growth, testosterone does not cause it. Recent studies suggest that it's actually elevated estrogen levels that increase a man's risk of prostate cancer.

Ligands increase levels of the phytoestrogens (plant estrogens) enterolactone and enterodiol. These mild estrogens block the stimulatory effect of harsher estrogens that lead to an increased risk of cancer in both men and women.

They also smooth out the hormonal swings associated with peri-menopause, thereby reducing peri-menopausal symptoms such as difficulty sleeping, mood swings, breast pain, fluid retention, "brain fog" and so on.

Ligands also help women who are already past menopause. One study of menopausal women showed that 4 tbsp of ground flaxseed daily (admittedly, a relatively high dose) reduced the frequency and severity of hot flashes by over 50%. (J Soc Integr Oncol. 2007 Summer; 5(3):106-12).

I usually recommend 2 tbsp/day, but a woman troubled with hot flashes may want to try the higher dose. Build up to it, though. The high fiber content might cause some GI upset if you go to the higher dose all at once.

There are some other benefits to including flax seed in your diet, but I think that's enough to see why it's on my list of recommended foods.

You can buy either the whole seed or pre-ground flaxseed meal. I get the whole seed and recommend you do the same.

For one thing, the whole seed is less expensive than flax meal. More importantly, the nutrients in flaxseed deteriorate rather rapidly once the seed coat has been broken.

If you do select ground flaxseed over whole seed, look for it in a vacuum sealed package, keep it in the refrigerator and use it up fairly quickly.

You may hear some producers claim that their particular color seed has superior nutritional value. I'm not aware of any reliable studies supporting such claims and I suspect this is more of a marketing ploy than anything else.

You do need to grind the seed to break the seed coat so the nutrients become available. Otherwise the seed will just pass through you without much benefit.

To grind it, use one of the mills more commonly used to grind coffee. Get one to use only for flaxseed unless you enjoy a few coffee grounds on your breakfast cereal more than I do. (BTW – the brand highest rated by the folks at America's Test Kitchen is the Krups Fast Touch, which sells for about 18 bucks. I've used one just about everyday for over 10 years so I can recommend it.)

I usually add the ground seed to my breakfast cereal. You can also add it to yogurt, a smoothie, cottage cheese, salad or anything else that appeals to you. Sometimes I just grind it, mix it with water and drink it as a slurry. It tastes OK to me, but then I'm inclined to do odd things if I think they're good for me.

Some of the studies on flaxseed provide it in the form of a muffin. Although it generally is better not to heat oils, baking doesn't appear to destroy much of flax seed's nutrients and this is an acceptable approach.

I should mention one lab study on rats. In this study, the offspring of pregnant rats given very high does of flax seed had a slightly higher rate of birth defects. This was only one study done with rats and with very high doses. There has not been any equivalent risk shown in humans.

Nonetheless, prudence dictates that any pregnant woman should discuss using flax seed with her physicians. If she does decide to eat it, she should stay on the low dose side.

You can also find flaxseed oil in either capsule or liquid form. Again, because the isolated oil doesn't contain the fiber, ligands and other micronutrients of the whole seed I consider freshly ground flax seeds preferable.

If you do purchase the oil, keep it in a cool dark place. Refrigeration is best. Don't use it for cooking because heat rapidly destroys its beneficial qualities. A good way to use the liquid oil is in a salad dressing, either by itself or mixed with olive oil.

## Curries

Until I was in my 20s, I thought that a curry was anything you made with the rather bland "curry powder" sold in most supermarkets in the 1950s. It wasn't until I bought a cookbook called The Vegetarian Epicure that I learned that the term 'curry' actually refers to a highly variable combination of spices and cooking methods.

Curries are a staple of the Indian diet but their exact nature varies wildly from region to region, town to town and even family to family.

Curries have become more popular in this country as Americans have become more adventurous in their eating patterns. I like curries for two reasons: they taste delicious and they're great for your health.

In the same way you can think of different colored vegetables as having a different variety of micro nutrients present, you can think of various spices and herbs as being concentrated forms of yet another wide array of nutrients for your body.

One example of why curries have come to the attention of Western researchers is the low incidence of Alzheimer's disease in India and Asian countries where curries are a common part of the diet. Researchers postulate that compounds in curry spices have anti-inflammatory effects and can slow the development of the amyloid plaques characteristic of Alzheimer's disease

Much of this research focuses on the spice turmeric and one of its components, curcumin. However curries contain a wide variety of other spices such as cumin, cardamom, coriander, garlic, ginger, etc. All of these have potential health benefits of their own.

As always, I think its best to get most of your nutrients from you diet. Curries are an excellent way to get a wide range of potentially helpful micronutrients in a way that tastes delicious. It's okay to take a turmeric supplement but it sure won't taste as good as a nice curry.

# 7 SUPPLEMENT SUGGESTIONS

To repeat myself, the most important aspect of nutrition is a healthy diet. Taking a multiple vitamin along with a donut doesn't make that a healthy meal.

On the other hand, I do think that supplements help many people. Some of my colleagues disagree. They believe that supplements aren't necessary. My belief is that while they may not be completely necessary in the sense that we can't survive without them, they have significant health benefits when properly used.

I think of supplements as insuring that we're getting enough of what we need everyday.

Also, it's becoming clear that we don't really know what levels of nutrients are really optimal. There's a big difference between the amount of a vitamin necessary to prevent an obvious nutritional disease such as scurvy or rickets and the amount that supports optimum vitality, not to mention wound healing.

In this section I'm going to begin by mentioning a few supplements that I think are particularly beneficial for wound healing. After that, I'll mention some supplements that may not be directly related to wound healing but that I believe can be beneficial for many people. I'll try to indicate the circumstances in which these supplements may be of help.

## High Potency Multivitamin

A general multivitamin mineral combination will ensure that you have at least some of most of the recognized vitamins and minerals. Most manufacturers try to include a high percentage of the current recommended daily value. This is fine, but many nutritionists and natural health experts argue that the daily values are woefully inadequate in many situations.

This controversy isn't going to be settled anytime soon so you are really going to have to use your own best judgment. I'll give you some ideas and tell you what I do but ultimately you'll have to decide for yourself.

To give you an idea of the products out there, here's the packaging label from a name brand multiple vitamin:

**Centrum® Ultra Men's Tablets**

Vitamin A 3,500 IU

Vitamin C 90 mg

Vitamin E 45 IU

Vitamin D 600 IU

Vitamin E 45 IU

Vitamin K 60 mcg

Thiamin 1.2 mg

Riboflavin 1.3 mg

Niacin 16 mg

Vitamin $B_6$ 2 mg

Folic Acid 200 mcg

Vitamin $B_{12}$ 6 mcg

Biotin 40 mcg

Pantothenic Acid 15 mg

Calcium 210 mg

Iron 8 mg

Phosphorus 20 mg

Iodine 150 mcg

Magnesium 100 mg

Zinc 11 mg

Selenium 100 mcg

Copper 0.9 mg

Manganese 2.3 mg

Chromium 35 mcg

Molybdenum 50 mcg

Chloride 72 mg

Potassium 80 mg

Boron 150 mcg

Nickel 5 mcg

Silicon 2 mg

Tin  10  mcg

Vanadium  10  mcg

Lycopene  600  mcg

This is a reasonable product, but it does have a little bit of what is referred to as "pixie dusting" going on. Pixie dusting is when manufactures include a trivial amount of a substance so they can claim additional benefits for their product.

In this case you'll note that the vitamin is labeled as "Centrum Men's Ultra Tablets". This implies that it contains some nutrients of particular benefit for men. In this regard, it does contain lycopene, which as I mentioned before, helps with prostate health. However, it only contains 600 **mcg** of lycopene. Studies that I've read on the benefits of lycopene generally look at doses on the range of 25 **mg**. There are 1000 mcg in 1 mg, which means that this product would have to contain 25,000 mcg of lycopene (not 600) to legitimately claim the benefits shown in those studies.

The same goes for boron. Centrum contains 150 **mcg**. The dose I recommend is 1 – 3 **mg**.

There's nothing wrong with getting the extra 600 mcg of lycopene or 150 mcg of boron from this tablet. Just don't expect that you gain the optimal amount of an ingredient because it's listed on the label.

Also be aware that manufacturers often charge a hefty premium for including the pixie dust. It's usually best to avoid these products for that reason.

By the way, you can easily get 25 mg of lycopene by drinking a glass of tomato juice. Salsa and tomato sauce are other good sources.

I don't intend to pick on Centrum by using it as my example. As I said, it's a decent product. However they clearly are interested in marketing and you may be able to get similar levels from a low cost generic, especially if you skip the pixie dust.

If you want to try "high dose" supplements, here are the dosages some experts suggest:

## High Dose Supplement Levels


A    2500 − 15,000 IU

Thiamine (B1) 25−100 mg

Riboflavin （B2） 25-50 mg

Niacin （B3） 50-200 mg

B6 10-50 mg

B12 600-1000 mcg

C 500-1000 mg

D 1000 - 2000 mg

E 400 IU

Folic acid （folate） 400-800 mcg （This is especially important for women of child-bearing age - taking folic acid dramatically reduces the risk of neural tube birth defects）.

Biotin 500 mcg

Pantothenic acid 3006—mg

There are a few premium products that will have those doses. If you can afford them they're fine to take, but not necessary. I've listed sources I trust on my website so the info remains up to date.

For the purposes of wound healing, take a solid general purpose multiple vitamin and mineral complex

103

and then take separate doses of select supplements that I'm going to recommend now.

## Vitamin C

Vitamin C is crucial for wound healing and scar formation. You've probably heard stories about how scurvy was endemic among sailors in the early days of long sea voyages without fresh provisions until the British discovered they could prevent it by issuing a ration of limes regularly.

The recommended daily value of vitamin C is 60 mg. While that's enough to prevent scurvy, I'm not sure it's optimal for wound healing.

At the wound center, we usually recommend higher doses 250 — 500 mg two or more times a day. Vitamin C is water soluble and readily excreted in the urine so I think it's advisable to take more than one dose a day to maintain consistently elevated levels.

By the way, some of my colleagues who are skeptical about the use of high doses of vitamins like to say that "the only thing they do is make expensive urine" because many are excreted in the urine the same way vitamin C is. My answer to them is to ask if they think that the only thing penicillin does is make expensive urine as well. 80% of penicillin is excreted unchanged in the urine. That doesn't mean it doesn't have important therapeutic effects as it passes through.

As a historical note, in the early years of WWII penicillin was in such demand and the supply was so short that health care workers collected the urine of patients who were receiving it so the penicillin could be isolated, purified and reused. ( Odd, the things I remember from my pharmacology class so many years ago. )

## Vitamin D

Vitamin D has deservedly received a lot of attention recently. Years ago, we believed that it's main importance was in calcium metabolism and bone formation. We now know that it plays a vital role in over 22,000 ( and counting ) metabolic pathways. Vitamin D is crucial for healthy immune function.

At the same time that we're realizing just how important vitamin D is, we're also discovering that a large percent of the population is deficient. Some surveys found that over 85% of the population living in climates north of Philadelphia have inadequate levels of vitamin D.

It's fair to call vitamin D "the sunshine vitamin" because sunlight stimulates vitamin D production in the skin. People in cold northern climates with short winter days obviously don't get much sun exposure for a good part of the year.

Also, concern about the risk of skin cancer and premature aging of the skin has made people much more likely to avoid the sun and to use a potent sunscreen when they are outside.

I won't bore you with my current recommendations about the use of sunscreen. I'll simply suggest that you take 1000 to 2000 units of vitamin D a day. This dosage is generally accepted as safe for anyone.

Personally, I take more in the winter when colds are endemic and I get virtually no sun exposure.

If you want to be more precise in the dose you take, it is possible to measure your blood levels of vitamin D (it's measured as 25-hydroxy vitamin D).

Although I routinely recommend getting levels checked to my patients and I think it's a great idea, I have to admit I never had mine checked until recently. When I did, I found that my level was right where I wanted it: 59 ng/ml. It's of note that at the time I was taking 7,000 units of vitamin D a day – 2,000 in the high-potency multiple vitamin I take and an additional 5,000 as a separate supplement. That's high dose supplementation, but less probably wouldn't have been adequate.

I suggest you aim for a level between 40 and 80 ng/ml. Most labs report levels greater than 20 as normal, but I don't believe that's optimal.

To further encourage you to supplement with vitamin D, you should know that low levels are associated with increased rates of multiple cancers. This may be because of vitamin D's importance for immune function. If you're dealing with cancer, levels closer to 80 are probably a good idea. However don't go overboard. Stay below 100.

There was considerable publicity given to the fact that the Food and Nutrition Board recently changed their Recommended Daily Allowance (RDA) for vitamin D. While raising it to 600 units/day was a step in the right direction, many researchers seriously interested in nutrition consider this recommendation completely inadequate. Since I'm taking a few thousand units of vitamin D daily myself I think you know which side of the debate I'm on.

In sum, I suggest that If you live in the north, or live in the south and don't get out in the sun much, you should assume you are deficient unless you've had your blood level checked to prove that you aren't. It's prudent to take a vitamin D supplement until you get your blood level checked.

## Whey Protein

Many people have trouble getting the increased protein they need for wound healing from their diet. Whey protein is a high quality protein derived from milk that can help. It is usually available as a powder.

Milk is mostly （87%） water. The 13% of solids in milk consist of fat, lactose and protein in roughly equal amounts, along with much smaller amounts of minerals.

That means roughly 4% of a glass of milk is protein. Milk protein is 80% casein and 20% whey.

Cheese is made from the casein and fat portion of milk. Whey is the liquid left over. Whey protein is isolated from the liquid whey in a variety of ways. The processing usually begins with passing the whey through a series of filters to remove some of the lactose and remaining fats.

At this point the water can be removed, resulting in whey protein concentrate. Or the manufacturer can pass the filtered liquid through an ion exchange tower. This further purifies the protein. When the water is removed now, the result is whey protein isolate.

Using enzymes and/or acids it is possible to break the whey down further into peptides. This product is whey protein hydrolysates.

These are all reasonable products but there are differences.

Whey contains biological components (beta-lactoglobulin, alpha-lactalbumin, glycomacropeptide, immunoglobulins and lactoferrin among others) that support immune function. Lactoferrin in particular seems to have anti-bacterial, anti-fungal and anti-viral properties. It also supports the health of the intestinal linings.

Whey protein concentrate has a higher level of lactoferrin and other components than the other whey products. The extra processing involved in making whey isolates or hydrolysates removes most of the lactoferrin.

On the other hand, whey isolates have a higher and more consistent level of protein. They also are virtually lactose-free. Concentrates are low in lactose, but they sometimes have enough residual lactose to bother someone who is very lactose intolerant. In these cases, it's worth trying a whey isolate. Most people with even severe lactose intolerance can tolerate an isolate because the amount of residual lactose is so low.

Because hydrolysates are partially broken down already, they are absorbed more readily. Also they are good for people with food allergies because they are less likely to trigger an allergic reaction.

In terms of cost, whey protein concentrates are the least expensive. Whey protein isolates are in the middle and whey protein hydrolysates are the most expensive.

Whey protein contains all essential amino acids and is also high in branched chained amino acids. Branched chained amino acids are important in muscle metabolism and muscle cells can absorb them directly.

This is a long-winded explanation to lead to the point: whey protein powders are a convenient way to add high-quality protein to your diet.

The powders usually come with a scoop to indicate the portion size which is usually between 15 g and 25 g of protein (the package will tell you what it is for a given product).

I usually recommend a serving once or twice a day between meals for most people dealing with a wound.

Whey protein powders are widely available because they are extremely popular with athletes, especially bodybuilders. GNC (a national chain of stores selling vitamins and supplements ) usually has a major section of their stores devoted to offering various whey protein products. Don't be put off by the fact that a lot of them will have images of hyper-developed bodybuilders on the package. Focus on what's in the package.

For most wound situations I recommend a whey concentrate or combination of concentrate and isolate. I like to include the concentrate because it reduces cost and also because of the higher levels of lactoferrin it contains.

Someone with extreme lactose intolerance may not tolerate a concentrate. In that case they should try a pure isolate.

For wound healing, I don't think the added expense of an hydrolysate is worth it. Its main advantage is that it is very rapidly absorbed and unlikely to trigger a food allergy. Athletes like to use this form of whey protein after workouts with the idea that rapid absorption provides branched chain amino acids to the muscles at the time when they're most likely to use it for growth. You don't need that rapid absorption for wound healing. In addition, isolates are virtually devoid of lactoferrin so you miss some of the immune boosting benefits.

You also don't need to bother with products that have additional ingredients, such as creatine, designed for athletes. Nor do I suggest that you use the so-called meal replacement powders. The most cost effective approach is to get a straightforward whey protein product.

As I mentioned, whey protein powders are widely available. I already told you about GNC. Some grocery stores will have them in their natural foods section. Health food stores carry them as well. Although they don't have as large of a selection, big-box stores such as BJ's often will have whey protein powder at a good price.

The largest selection and best prices I've seen are on the Internet at the site www.bodybuilding.com. You may want to buy some small packages of protein locally to make sure it agrees with you. If it does, you can comparison shop online.

Many people use Boost or Ensure or similar products as meal replacements or a dietary supplement. These products are okay, but I'm not a huge fan. The fats and carbohydrates they contain aren't particularly high quality and their protein levels are low.

On the other hand, if someone is having trouble eating for whatever reason but likes these products they are certainly much better than nothing. If you are going to use them, you can improve the nutritional profile by adding some whey protein. Thin it with a bit of water if necessary.

## Arginine

Arginine is a unique amino acid necessary for wound healing. As you may recall from earlier, we can classify amino acids as being essential (we need to get them from our diet) or non-essential (our body can produce them from other amino acids).

That's a useful classification, but it's not the whole story. There are some amino acids that are in between. We call these conditionally essential or semi-essential. This means that while we have the potential to produce the amino acid, sometimes the need exceeds our ability to synthesize it. In this situation, our diet needs to contain enough of the conditionally essential amino acid to meet the extra requirement.

Arginine is such an amino acid. In a normal maintenance situation where we are going through life without any major issues, arginine is not essential. If needed, internal production could meet our needs.

However, in certain situations the demand for arginine exceeds our internal ability to provide it. That's when it becomes essential and we need to be certain we include it in our diet.

Wound healing is one such situation. Arginine is a precursor of the material that eventually becomes collagen, the stuff scar tissue is made of. This means that if you don't have enough arginine you're not going to be able to form scars optimally.

Several studies have shown that arginine enhances both healing and immune function in people with wounds.


## Glutamine


Glutamine is another non-essential amino acid that can become conditionally essential in some situations – like stress and wound healing.

Glutamine is important for muscle growth and also has antioxidant properties. Glutamine is an important energy source for the cells that line the GI tract and multiple cells in the immune system.

Most studies have been in burn patients and acutely ill surgical patients. The results have been mixed, with some showing no benefit and others showing that it does help. These studies also often use glutamine given intravenously rather that orally because of the severity of the illness of the patients being treated.

Some studies looking at experimental wounds and chronic pressure wounds in outpatients have shown a positive result from supplementation with a combination of arginine, glutamine and another compound called HMB. That combination is available in a commercially available product called Juven. Juven is a good product but it is somewhat pricey. You can get most of the benefit for less buying arginine and glutamine separately.

With regards to glutamine, if a person's nutritional status is questionable or healing seems stalled, I recommend 5 g 1 – 3 times/day. If I had to choose between arginine and glutamine, I'd pick arginine first, then add glutamine.

As a side note, some people think that taking glutamine at bed time can increase growth hormone levels (a good thing – higher levels of growth hormone increase muscle mass and decrease body fat). If you are going to take glutamine, consider taking a dose in the morning and another before bed.

# Fish Oil

I went on for quite a while about fish oil in the section on fats so I won't belabor the point here other than to repeat the recommendation to take one or two grams of fish oil with breakfast and dinner.

# Glucosamine

Many people use glucosamine to relieve arthritis, and it is helpful for that. However it is also a useful supplement to support wound healing.

Fibroblasts, the cells that form scar tissue, secrete hyaluronic acid in the early stages of wound healing. Hyaluronic acid in turn stimulates the attraction of more fibroblasts and the multiplication of epithelial cells. (Check the appendix if you want more information on the stages of wound healing.)

Glucosamine is the substrate for the production of hyaluronic acid. If there isn't enough glucosamine available production of hyaluronic acid will be less than optimal.

I'm not aware of any human studies that definitely prove glucosamine helps wound healing. On the other hand, we know from extensive studies on glucosamine in the treatment of arthritis that it is an extremely safe supplement to take. For this reason, I consider glucosamine in the class of things that "won't hurt and might help".

If you do want to try glucosamine, animal studies suggest that the production of hyaluronic acid and other glycosaminoglycans is highest in the early stages of wound healing, peaking at five days. This suggests that the most appropriate time to supplement is in the early stages of wound healing.

It also suggests that it might be helpful to supplement with glucosamine prior to and immediately after scheduled surgery. The usual recommended dose is 500 mg 3 times per day.

## Zinc

Wound healing requires adequate levels of zinc, but supplementation is helpful only if a person is deficient and not getting enough in their diet.

The official RDA is around 11 mg/day for adults. Zinc is one supplement where you need to be certain not to go overboard. Too much zinc in your diet interferes with copper absorption, leading to copper deficiency.

Also, paradoxically, too much zinc might hinder wound healing. These problems can occur with a steady intake as low as 25 my/day. Most people will tolerate significantly more, but it's reasonable to be cautious at the high end.

Zinc is present in many foods. Most people get the majority of their zinc from beef, which has over 8 mg in four ounces. The food with the highest concentration of zinc are oysters, which have 75 mg in a half dozen.

It's difficult to assess whether or not zinc status is adequate clinically, but research studies suggest that 35% – 45% of adults 60 years of age or older may be zinc deficient.

As a practical matter, we often recommend that someone with a problem wound supplements with zinc for at least a few weeks. We especially recommend this for older people and anyone with pre-existing nutrition problems.

The dose we recommend is 10 - 15 mg/day. People with chronic diarrhea, pre-existing malnutrition or absorption problems may need significantly more.

If you're taking a multivitamin and mineral combination, be sure to see if contains zinc and reduce the amount you take as a separate supplement accordingly. Some high potency brands frequently have a lot of zinc in them. In fact, the brand I usually take provides 35 mg/day. I certainly don't need to be taking any more.

## Magnesium

While magnesium isn't crucially involved in wound healing, it is a crucial mineral. Magnesium is the second most common mineral within the cells and is involved in many metabolic processes. It is very important for nerve conduction and muscle contraction. In particular, it helps stabilize heart rhythms.

Also, although calcium gets most of the attention, magnesium is important for bone strength as well.

Many of us don't get enough magnesium in our diets, and we're more likely to become deficient as we age. In addition, many drugs, such as diuretics, lower magnesium levels even more.

Lots of studies suggest the importance of magnesium. For example, nurses participating in the Nurses' Health Study with the highest levels of magnesium in their diet and in their serum had the lowest rate of sudden cardiac death.

Other studies confirm a beneficial influence of magnesium on heart disease. Given the importance of magnesium for smooth nerve conduction and muscle contraction this isn't surprising.

Magnesium has other benefits as well. It helps small blood vessels relax so it is helpful in modulating high blood pressure. Also, I've had many people get relief from night cramps and "restless leg syndrome" after they started taking magnesium.

I suggest supplementing with 250 mg – 500 mg of magnesium a day, taking at least part of the dose at bedtime.

# Co-enzyme Q10

Coenzyme Q10 (Co Q-10) is another supplement that isn't specific for wound healing but I often recommend it to people at the clinic. Many people who have problems healing wounds also have problems that Co Q-10 can help with.

Co Q10 is a compound found naturally in the part of the cell called the mitochondria. Mitochondria are the energy producing parts of the cell. You can think of them as a cell's power stations.

In addition to helping produce energy, Co Q-10 also works as an antioxidant, always a good thing to have around. Rust is a form of oxidation and the equivalent can happen in our bodies if we don't have enough antioxidants.

Another name for Co Q-10 that you hear less frequently is ubiquinone because coenzyme Q10 is found in every cell in the body (it's "ubiquitious").

Co Q-10 levels tend to decrease gradually with age. Also, very importantly some commonly prescribed drugs lower levels even further.

Supplementing with coenzyme Q10 can help lower cholesterol, lower high blood pressure, and strengthen the heart in congestive heart failure. Since Co Q-10 is very safe and very well tolerated, I think you can see why this is a useful supplement to consider taking.

It's especially important that anyone taking a drug of the statin class ( Lipitor, etc. ) seriously consider supplementing with coenzyme Q-10. While it's best to lower cholesterol to healthy levels without resorting to statins, sometimes they are necessary. Unfortunately, as with any drug, the use of statins comes with a risk of side effects.

Statins work by blocking the production of cholesterol. However they also block the production of other compounds including coenzyme Q-10. This may be the mechanism that causes the muscle pain and liver damage often associated with the use of statins. In my opinion, anyone who has to take a statin drug should take Co Q-10 along with it.

As a general supplement, I suggest 30 mg to 100 mg of coenzyme Q-10 daily. For people with congestive heart failure, coronary artery disease or taking statin drugs I recommend 100 mg twice a day.

Co Q-10 is not very readily absorbed. It is fat soluble so taking it with a little bit of dietary fat helps with absorption. Since I recommend fish oil capsules for just about everybody, I suggest people taking CoQ 10 take it along with their fish oil.

Some manufacturers promote a form of Co Q-10 known as ubiquinol (vs. ubiquinone − standard Co-Q 10). They claim that this form of Co Q-10 is absorbed more readily and has greater biologic effectiveness. This may well be true, but I haven't seen independent evidence to prove it.

Recently, some labs offer tests for Co Q-10 levels. If I had serious heart disease or felt I had to take statin drugs I would definitely have my levels checked and supplement accordingly.

# Probiotics

While not directly related to wound healing, I definitely want to mention probiotics in this section because many people dealing with chronic wounds will require antibiotics to treat infection at some point. In that situation it's extremely important to take probiotics in one form or another.

Probiotics refer to beneficial bacteria. While we often think of bacteria as the bad guys, the fact is we coexist with them routinely. Most are harmless and many are actually beneficial.

When we take antibiotics we upset the natural order of things. As one of the nurses at the wound center likes to tell our patients, "Antibiotics are dumb. They don't just go to the infection, they kill everything."

When you have lots of healthy bacteria competing for nutrients disease causing bacteria have trouble getting a foothold. Taking antibiotics changes that balance. It gives the true bad guys a chance to take over. Clinically, this shows up as diarrhea. Sometimes people develop an invasive infection on the colon (colitis) that can even be life threatening. Clostridium difficile (c diff.) infections are notorious for this.

Healthy bacteria also compete with yeast for nutrients. This means that reducing the population of healthy bacteria increases the possibility of developing a yeast infection. This most commonly presents as a yeast infection of the throat (thrush) or as a vaginal yeast infection in women.

Replenishing normal bacteria colonies by taking probiotics reduces the chances of these problems developing. It doesn't eliminate them completely, but it does put the odds in your favor.

Probiotics are available over-the-counter at pharmacies and in health food stores. Look for a brand containing several different bacterial strains and a guaranteed minimal bacteria count.

You can also look for the addition of something called fructo-oligosaccharide. Fructo-oligosaccharide is one of a class of compounds known as prebiotics. Prebiotics are foods that we can't digest and absorb but that can nourish healthy bacteria. Another benefit of ground flax seed is that its fiber serves as a prebiotic.

You can also get healthy bacteria by eating yogurt with active cultures. In keeping with my recommendation to base your nutrition on wholesome foods, I think it's best to use both yogurt and probiotics. Use non-fat or low-fat yogurt. Add fruit and sweeten it yourself. I'm not a big fan of artificial sweeteners but I do prefer them to all the added sugar in many yogurts. If just adding berries or fruit isn't sweet enough, it's better to sweeten your yogurt with a herb known as stevia. Stevia has been used as a sweetener in Central and South America. The crushed leaf of the whole herb has a bit of aftertaste that I never liked. However, a specific extract (rabaudioside A) is now available as a food additive in the U.S. and this extract tastes much better. It is commonly available under several brand names such as Truvia, Sweet Leaf, PureVia, etc. You can probably find it in the sweetener section of your local supermarket.

Stevia has no effect on blood sugar and in fact may even improve glucose tolerance. It doesn't cook well, but it works fine to sweeten coffee and tea.

Take yogurt and/or probiotics twice a day whenever you're on antibiotics and for at least a couple of weeks afterwards. Take the probiotics with meals, and don't take them at the same time as the antibiotics.

# Other Supplements

There are other supplements, including herbs, that I recommend for other problems. The list here includes the ones I recommend most often to people with problem wounds. Things like alpha lipoic acid, selenium, milk thistle and more definitely have their place but describing them all here wound be somewhat of a digression. If you are interested in learning more about other supplements you can visit my web site at http://www.jfmccaffreymd.com.

# 8 SUMMING IT ALL UP

We've covered a lot of material and a lot of details. I hope I haven't made it seem too confusing. It doesn't have to be. Let's go over things again in a quick summary to emphasize the main points.

Nutrition is a key to good health in general and wound healing in particular. Your food provides the raw materials that allow the miracle of healing to proceed. Getting enough food in terms of calories isn't an issue for most people in this country but getting appropriate nutrients definitely is.

To sum up the suggestions I've made:

- Remember that you set the foundation for healing by eating healthy food
- Wound healing increases protein needs. Emphasize the lean sources of protein mentioned here
- Eat a wide array of fruits and vegetables
- Include healthy fat in your diet
- Avoid sugars and refined foods
- Consider supplementing with: whey protein, fish oil, a multivitamin, vitamin C, vitamin D, magnesium, arginine, glutamine, glucosamine and zinc

- If you have to take antibiotics, be sure to also take yogurt and/or probiotics.

As I mentioned in the beginning, eating the way I suggest in this book is a good idea whether you have a wound or not. The "secret" to staying healthy and living a vital life really isn't all that secret: eat a healthy diet (and really, you don't need me to tell you what that is), don't put poisons in your body (cigarettes, excess alcohol, etc.), consider taking a few supplements, exercise appropriately, maintain a healthy attitude and manage stress effectively.

Simple, isn't it? Yet easier said than done. Be easy about it. Small, steady changes in the right direction do add up.

If you're struggling to heal a wound, I hope the information here helps you heal. More than that, I hope it helps you live a vital, vibrant life. Stay well.

# APPENDIX

# PHASES OF WOUND HEALING

It doesn't take much reflection to realize how miraculous wound healing is. Consider a "simple" cut. Let's say you're working in the garden and get a deep scratch on your forearm or nick yourself as you're cutting twine. One moment you're going along with no injury and the next your body's outer line of protection, your skin, has been breached and tissue damaged. This triggers an immediate and automatic response that begins immediately and will continue for years.

To make it easier to understand, we describe four phases of healing: inflammatory, migratory, proliferative and late remodeling. In reality, healing is a continuum and we're really only beginning to understand what is going on and how the body orchestrates it. However, here's the general time line:

Inflammatory (1-4 days)

Migratory (4 days to 6 weeks)

Proliferative   5 days to 3 weeks

Late remodeling 3 weeks to 1 year

Let's look at these phases in more detail.

## Inflammatory Phase

Immediately after an acute injury, the first order of business is to stop the bleeding. To this end, platelets clump together to plug severed capillaries. At the same time, they release chemicals that cause blood vessels to constrict and also trigger numerous cascades of chemical reactions.  One such cascade results in the formation of blood clots.

While this is happening, the damaged cells release chemical signals that attract specialized white blood cells to the area, the most populous of which at this phase are polymorphonuclear neutrophils (PMNs). Within an hour, these cells are active within the wound, killing bacteria and clearing debris.

PMNs are most active in the first few days after injury. Over this period of time other white blood cells, monocytes, migrate to wound. These cells are attracted by chemicals released by the injured cells and platelets. As monocytes move from the capillaries into the wound they transform into macrophages, cells that can engulf bacteria, bits of damaged tissue and dead PMNs. They also release a number of enzymes that help clean the wound as well as additional growth factors that stimulate the further progression of wound healing.

If wound healing is progressing smoothly, the inflammatory phase starts to subside after 3 −5 days. At this point, the wound should be relatively clean and the number of neutrophils and macrophages decreasing. The inflammatory phase is now subsiding and the migratory phase becomes dominate.

## Migratory Phase

During the migratory phase, new blood vessels begin to grow into the damaged area. Very importantly, cells called fibroblasts migrate in as well. Fibroblasts are

133

the cells that lay down collagen, the material that scars are made of and that gives a healed wound its strength.

Epithelium is the outer layer of skin. Cells from this layer also migrate over the wound at this time.

In short, a lot of the specialized cells needed for healing move into the area of the wound during the migratory phase.

## Proliferative Phase

The proliferative phase generally begins about day 5. This is a phase when things really start to happen. Production of collagen by the fibroblasts and scar development rapidly increases as healing kicks into high gear.

A fascinating process that also begins during the proliferative phase is wound contraction. Specialized cells called myofibroblasts begin to appear at the wound edge, probably developing from regular fibroblasts.

Myofibroblasts differ in that they have microfilaments within them that are very much like similar strands in muscle cells. These cells have the ability to contract. In doing so they pull the wound edges together. Depending on how tight the skin is, wounds can contract at up to 0.75 mm/day.

As an aside, don't all these reactions taking place and cells changing from one form to another as needed strike you as miraculous? It does me.

Getting back to the phases of wound healing...

The amount of collagen in the wound increases rapidly during the first 3 weeks, then levels off. At this point the late remodeling phase begins.

## Remodeling and Late Remodeling

During remodeling cells become less numerous in the wound, old collagen is broken down and new collagen is laid down along the lines of stress. This increases the strength of the wound. Additional chemical bonds develop between strands of collagen that further increase the strength of the healed wound.

135

At 1 week, a wound has very little strength. It's remarkable that skin stays together when we take stitches out after a week or so. Even after a month, the wound will only be about ½ as strong as it will be at a year. At 6 weeks that increases to about ¾ of its eventual strength.

After the first two months or so, the rate of remodeling then slows dramatically, but continues for years. You have probably noticed yourself that scars from an injury you had years ago look much different today than they did one month after the injury. I certainly have had this experience: I burned the inside of my arm during residency and it healed with a scar that was very noticeable for years. Today you can hardly tell where the burn was. That's remodeling at work.

This outline only hints at the complexity of interactions required to organize all this. To give you some idea, I alluded to chemical mediators. These include things having names like platelet-derived growth factor, transforming growth factor, metalloproteinases, fibroblast growth factor, tumor necrosis factor and on and on. The deeper researches look, the more they find.

For example, we usually refer to collagen as if it was one chemical, but it turns out there are at least 18 different types of collagen.

Fortunately, we don't have to have conscious awareness of every known nuance of wound healing for our wounds to heal. That miracle happens by itself. But it helps if we do what we can to create the best possible circumstances for healing. Part of that is making sure our bodies have the raw materials they need available. That's what proper nutrition and this book are about.

# DISCLAIMER

This book is for informational purposes only. The information provided here should not be construed as personal medical advice or instruction.

The Content is not intended to be a substitute for professional medical advice, diagnosis, or treatment.

Always seek the advice of your physician or other qualified health provider with any questions you may have regarding a medical condition.

Never disregard professional medical advice or delay in seeking it because of something you have read here.

We do not recommend or endorse or guarantee any specific products, procedures, opinions, or other information that may be mentioned in this book.
Use of the information here is solely at your own risk. The publisher is not responsible for errors or omissions.

Joseph F. McCaffrey MD, FACS

# ABOUT THE AUTHOR

Dr. McCaffrey is a general and vascular surgeon with over 30 years experience caring for people with complex surgical issues. He has a long-standing interest in the important contribution factors such mental attitude, stress management and nutrition make to a person's overall well-being. His professional goal is to help people live vital lives.

He currently limits his practice to wound care and hyperbaric medicine.

Joseph F. McCaffrey MD, FACS

# Index

## A

## B

## C

## D

# E

empty calories, 11, 25, 27

# F

fish oil, iv, 23, 72, 73, 76, 77, 78, 90, 119, 126, 131
Flaxseed, 89, 90, 91
fructo-oligosaccharide, 128

# G

Garlic, 83
Glutamine, 117, 118

# H

hot flashes, 93
hydrostatic underwater weighing, 15

# I

immune system, 8, 13, 90, 118
immunoglobulins, 112

# L

ligands, 74, 90, 91, 92, 95
Lipitor, 125
lycopene, 87, 103, 104
lycopenes, 87

# M

macronutrient, 19, 25
magnesium, 122, 123, 131
Michael Pollan, 4
micronutrients, 27, 78, 79, 95, 97

# V

Vegetables, 79
Vitamin C, 101, 106
vitamin D, iv, 108, 109, 110, 131

# W

Whey protein, 110, 111, 112, 113

# Y

yeast infection, 128
yogurt, 67, 68, 75, 94, 128, 129

# Z

zinc, 121, 122, 131

www.ingramcontent.com/pod-product-compliance
Lightning Source LLC
Chambersburg PA
CBHW070136290526
45789CB00002B/503